The Road to Ultimate Peace: My Parents' Cancer Diagnosis, Treatment, Fight and My Role in Their Care

By

Derick Hendricks

Dedicated to the loving memory of my parents: Elmo Hendricks, Sr. and Eleanor Chesterfield Hendricks

Table of Contents

Other books by Derick Hendricks

The Confusion
Leaf from Round the Field

Published by Lulu

Prologue

This book is not a scholarly piece of work. In no way, is it meant to be an academic text. On the contrary, this essay is an account of my parents' cancer diagnosis, treatment, fight and how I dealt with it. In addition to documenting some circumstances, which were related to their illness, and how I reacted to them, my wish is for this literature to positively touch the life of at least one person, who experienced the horrors that I did, when I learned that my parents had become cancer patients, and to provide some sort of hope and peace of mind to the aforementioned individual. Accordingly, my intention for this book is to serve the following two purposes: 1. To keep a record of an important phase in the lives of my parents and myself and 2. To help other individuals who may be or may have been in a similar situation as we were.

Part 1

The Beginning

Chapter 1

My Father's Diagnosis and Treatment

The week of June 14, 2005 was supposed to be a celebratory time for me and my wife because, eight years earlier, on Saturday, June 14, 1997, Carol-Ann and I were married in St. Thomas, U.S. Virgin Islands. We decided to spend our eighth anniversary in Ocean City, Maryland. Although we did travel to Ocean City, and we did observe our anniversary, the period was marked with much uncertainty and fear because of the unexpected news that my mother had given me. I can clearly remember my mother's words, the instability of her voice, my reaction, where I was when I got the message, and everything else about that day. Carol-Ann and I had been driving for a couple hours to our destination; listening to the radio; talking about the weekend's plans; our marriage; etc. While cruising along the highway, my cell phone rang, and it was my mother on the other end of the line. After speaking to her for a few minutes, the tone of her voice lowered to a near whisper and a tremble. Then, she said, "Ummmm, Derick, I have something to tell you. Ummm, you know your father and I usually go to the doctor for checkups, right? Well, ummmm, your father had to give the doctor a specimen of his stool. They sent it away to study it, and, ummm, they found something." Those last three words-they found something-rippled through my mind like a raging fire. Although I did not know exactly what the words meant, I knew, for sure, that it was not good news based on the change in my mother's attitude and speech.

After I questioned her about what was found, she said, "They found cancer." Cancer. Wow. Although I was aware of family members and friends who were living with the disease, or who had died from it, my father was my closest relative who had been diagnosed with it. What a mind shocker. All I kept saying to myself was,

"Cancer? Cancer. Cancer? Damn. Damn. Damn." I don't know which one was

racing faster: my heart or my mind. As expected, my mother did not tell me too much

information about the situation, including the next step for my father, because the

doctor's conclusion was very recent. Shortly after she gave me the news, we concluded

our conversation on an optimistic and upbeat note. Despite our positive demeanor, I

was taken aback, sad, frightened, angry, and pessimistic about my father's prognosis.

Although I cannot prove it, I am sure that my mother felt the same way as I did. Once I

had disconnected the call, I shared the news with Carol-Ann. Like me, she was

shocked and sad after she learned of the cancer specialist's opinion. Immediately, she

began to cheer me up and advised me that the diagnosis did not necessarily mean that

my father would die. She assured me that it was not an automatic death sentence.

While my father was facing years of cancer treatment and recovery, she assured me

that he could beat the illness. Carol-Ann emphasized that I put my trust in God, pray

about the matter, and do my best to help with the entire situation. I listened to her

carefully and thanked her for her kindness and counseling. As I remained silent in the

car and peered through the window, I could not help but ask myself the following

questions: What would be next for my father? Would he suffer? How much longer

would he live? Was Carol-Ann correct when she said he could beat the disease? Only

time would tell.

As planned, Carol-Ann and I commemorated our eighth wedding

anniversary in Ocean City, Maryland. I did my best to enjoy myself and the significance of the milestone. However, to be sure, I was still upset and worried about my father's health. Although I attempted to shield my emotions from Carol-Ann, she was totally aware of my feelings and was understandable. Certainly, her words and deeds that weekend were commendable. Shortly after we returned to Baltimore, Maryland, I spoke to my mother, and she gave me additional information about my father's health. She reiterated what she had told me earlier that my father underwent his regular checkup; the doctor sent away a body sample; and the test results showed that my father had cancer. Subsequently, I was told by one of my brothers that our father had seen blood in his stool and alerted the primary care physician about it. Thereafter, the medical practitioner mailed away a specimen, and it was found to be cancerous.

To be sure this was grave news. Moreover, the matter became even more urgent when my mother told me that my father was scheduled to have emergency surgery immediately at the Roy L. Schneider (RLS) Hospital, and she wanted me to come home (St. Thomas) for it. She also wanted my oldest brother (Butch) to come to St. Thomas for the surgery. My third sibling, who is older than me and younger than my oldest brother, lived in St. Thomas. Consequently, my parents' three off springs were in St. Thomas for the operation. On the day of the medical procedure, my brothers, my mother, my maternal grandmother, and my great aunt-my father's aunt-were at the hospital with my father. Prior to my father being wheeled into the room, my mother asked my brothers and me to pray. I recall my oldest brother crying, while he was praying. This was a total shock to me because it was the first time that I had seen him shed tears. My other brother said an authoritative prayer that was characterized with much clarity, force, and enunciation. Clearly, his prayer also surprised me because I did not know he was so religious! My prayer was short and direct. Then, an employee came and gave my father, and the rest of us, instructions about what was to happen next. As the worker started to wheel my father into the emergency room, he kept smiling and looked optimistic about his new venture. His manner was not unusual because this was not out of his normal character. My mother kissed him, squeezed his hand, and then she started to cry. Upon seeing my mother crying and watching my father being taken to the operating room, I began crying silently. When I was about 12 years old, my father had fallen off of a roof and had broken his arm. Other than that accident, my father's cancer diagnosis and the anticipated surgery were the only other times that I had known him to be hospitalized or even sick. Consequently, I was emotional in the hospital. However, once I realized that no one was reacting to my sadness and aware of the fact that I had to show strength for my mother, I stopped shedding tears immediately.

The next couple hours felt like a century. By this time, my eldest brother's former girlfriend-she continued to stay in touch with my parents, and she is like a family member-was at the hospital with us. Additionally, my god mother-who was my mother's co-worker for several decades and friend-was also at the medical facility. We all sat in the waiting room and engaged in small talk. Every now and then, someone would look outside the room to see if the surgeon was walking down the hall to come and speak with us. Finally, the surgeon came and provided us with an update. He began by saying that the operation went well. The surgical team was able to remove the cancerous tumors from my father's colon. He continued; however, that the cancer had spread to the liver, and it was a stage four. Stage four. Wow. While I am not familiar with oncology and other matters related to cancer, the mere term "stage four" did not sound like good news. And I was correct. Thereafter, the physician explained the various levels of cancer, and he detailed for us exactly what the fourth stage of cancer meant. Very meticulously, he noted that the cancerous tumor was malignant, and it had metastasized to my father's liver. We asked the doctor a few questions, and he answered each one satisfactorily. Thereafter, he informed us that my father was in the recovery room, and he told us not to be alarmed by my father's appearance nor by the groans and moans that he would be making. The doctor explained that my father would not be able to respond to us physically or verbally, until after a couple hours, and that this was not out of the ordinary. Once the brief talk ended, my mother led the way down the hall to the recovery room. Everyone else followed, and I was the last person to enter the room. Before I saw my father, I noticed that my mother was sitting outside the room, and she was crying. Every now and then, she went in the room, touched my father, mumbled a few words, and then went back outside to weep while sitting. This was terrible to witness. Even though everyone was happy that the surgery was successful, we all knew that there was a major struggle ahead of us.

What was the next step for my father and his loved ones? He spent a few days in the hospital to recover and then went home. Prior to being discharged from the medical facility, the surgeon informed us that my father would have to undergo chemotherapy, in order to slow down (and possibly stop) the spread of the tumors. Chemotherapy. Chemo. Wow. Although I had heard the terms before, I did not know exactly how it would affect my father. To be sure, none of us, including the family patriarch, was certain about the treatment. Nevertheless, our fear and anxiety, to some extent, was eased after the surgeon explained that chemo patients responded differently to the medication. For instance, he noted, some people lose their hair, some individuals lose weight, and there are others who lose neither their hair nor their weight. Additionally, the doctor was adamant that he would not estimate how many months, years, or any other time period that my father would live after the cancer surgery. Along these lines, the doctor pointed out that he once had a patient, who did not lose any weight, and he recalled another one who lived for several years following her operation. While these were some positive statements from the medical practitioner, he cautioned us that all of our lives would forever be changed. This was a very accurate assessment.

My father was an electrician and a very hard worker. Anytime something needed to be done in and/or around the house, he would work on it. If he couldn't fix it, he would hire someone to do it. Of course, if the problem in the house was an electrical issue, he would solve the dilemma himself. Well, this would come to a complete stop, beginning in the fall of 2005. Accordingly, after a few weeks of recuperating from cancer surgery, the chemotherapy sessions began.

It should be noted that in 1985, my oldest brother moved to Florida from St. Thomas. Fifteen years later, on July 13, 2000, my wife and I relocated from St. Thomas to Chesapeake, Virginia. As a result, when my father's illness was revealed, my parents were the sole persons, who were living in the house, with the exception of my older sibling and his family, who lived on the first floor of the edifice. Prior to 2005, I had not returned to St. Thomas until December of 2004, when I traveled there for my grandmother's 80th birthday celebration. Meanwhile, in August of 2002, I began a rigorous PhD program at Morgan State University in Baltimore, Maryland. However, following my father's diagnosis and surgery, I made it a priority to return to St. Thomas during the summer and Christmas breaks. Subsequently, I also made a trip home during the spring and Thanksgiving breaks. The duration of these visits ranged from one and a half weeks to one month.

When I went back to St. Thomas in 2005, my father did not look any different from when I had last seen him two years earlier and in 2004. Accordingly, in spring 2003, I boarded a Greyhound Bus, traveled to Miami, Florida, and surprised my parents, who were in that city to attend the wedding of my eldest brother's former girlfriend. This lady is the same person who had flown to St. Thomas for my father's surgery. It was the first time that I had seen my father since 2000, when my wife and I had relocated to Virginia. Although I noticed that my father had lost some weight, since 2003, I did not think too much about it. As noted previously, the following year, my wife and I traveled to St. Thomas-this was the first time that I had been to the land of my birth, since we had relocated in 2000-in order to attend my grandmother's 80th birthday party. Again, while my father did look thin, I was not alarmed by his physique. In retrospect, I can remember my mother telling me on the telephone that my father had lost weight; that he was looking skinnier; etc; however, no one-not my mother, my father, his siblings, my mother's siblings, and other friends and family members-raised any alarm. When my mother mentioned to her sister, a retired nurse who lives in New York, that my father did not look as physically fit as he was accustomed to, my aunt simply said, "Well, he is getting older. As a result, it is normal for him to lose the weight because it is part of the aging process." Meanwhile, my grandmother's reaction to the change in my father's body mass was merely, "Well, you know, he was never a fat person. He has always been a thin fellow." In hindsight, I wish that everyone, including my father, had taken a more proactive approach when we all observed that he was losing weight. Even more, I wish that my father's primary care physician had advised him to get a colonoscopy. Although my father regularly went to the doctor for examinations, including prostate exams, he never had a colonoscopy. While the past cannot be changed, as a human being, I still keep wondering, "Why? Why my father?" and I continue to wish that things were done differently. Nevertheless, as noted earlier, after he was diagnosed with colon cancer and began chemotherapy treatment, his life changed forever.

As noted earlier, my father was an electrician. Although he had retired from the Virgin Islands Port Authority, in 1991, he continued to do electrical work. Thus, after he had left government service, he spent more time enhancing his private electrical business and doing other tasks at home. Additionally, since 1991, my parents actively participated in my father's family reunion organization: the Hermon-Birch-Gibbs Family Reunion Committee. The club's highlight was taking a Caribbean cruise once every two years. To be sure, my parents traveled with the group on each one of the trips. I was fortunate enough to sail with the reunion group on two occasions: in 1991 and in 1993. Prior to the appearance of this monster, cancer, in our lives, other activities that my father was involved in included, grocery shopping, attending public fairs, and doing other daily chores. These types of events and others would come to an abrupt halt, beginning in the summer of 2005.

As noted previously, prior to the beginning of the chemo sessions, the lead surgeon briefed my father's loved ones about the therapy. He noted that my father would receive chemo every week, and that, based on how the medication worked, there would be periods when my father would get a break from the chemo. Because I did not know much about chemotherapy, I did a little research on the subject and found that the medicine is a catch 22. That is, while it kills the cancer cells, it also destroys white blood cells, which are necessary to do away with many sorts of infections. As a result, at the beginning of each week, my father would undergo one round of chemo and then, at the end of the week, he would receive an injection that would help to replenish his white blood cells. This cycle began shortly after the June 2005 operation, and it continued for the next few weeks. Initially, my father did not have any noticeable negative reactions from the chemotherapy. He continued to drive, complete household chores-like sweeping the floor, washing dishes, and vacuuming-and he was capable of cooking his own meals.

In the meantime, the method of how the chemo was given to my father was altered. Although my mother explained the new development to me, on many occasions, I was, and I still am a little confused about it. She noted that there came a point, eventually, when he was given an electronic device, which measured and/or monitored the chemo drugs in his system. The size of a fanny pack, he took the device with him where ever he went. My mother informed me that the apparatus would make beeping sounds whenever it needed to be re-fitted or re-energized. Once the small machine sounded off, one of my parents would call the hospital and let the medical staff know about it. Unsurprisingly, the arrangement was problematic, at times. For instance, I was told that, on many occasions, the device would wake my parents at night with the alert. Eventually, this method of my father using the electronic gadget was discontinued.

Later, physical changes began to appear, a few weeks into the chemo sessions. I can vividly recall the day when my mother told me of the chemo's ramifications. One morning, shortly after my parents had awaken, my father observed pieces of hair on his pillow. In shock, he turned to my mother and exclaimed to her: "What is that!?! Hair? Whose hair is that for? Mine!?!" For the first time, to my parents' perception, the chemo had attacked. While they both knew that the medicine eliminated the healthy white blood cells, to them, the sight of the hair on the pillow made my father's cancer even more real. In that moment, I am certain, all sorts of questions raced through my father's mind. Inquiries, such as, "Am I going to go bald? Will I have to wear a toupee?" were sure to have crossed his mind. To be sure, his concern impacted him mentally, more so than that of my mother and everyone else. Nonetheless, my father continued with his chemotherapy and did not complain about his new lifestyle.

Another change that resulted from my father having cancer regarded religion. A Moravian, he attended New Hernhut Moravian church, and my mother, a Lutheran, attended Frederick Evangelical Lutheran church. However, after my father's diagnosis and subsequent surgery, my mother began to accompany him to Moravian church. Although she never rescinded her membership, this was a major change for her because she attended Lutheran church every Sunday and was an active choir member there. In addition to weekly services, my mother went with him to Christmas and spring concerts, Bible study, picnics, and other actives that were held at the Moravian church. One more challenge that my father faced dealt with the availability of his medicine. Sometimes, the drugs were not available because they had not been shipped as scheduled from Puerto Rico. As everyone would realize, later, my father's hair loss, the inaccessibility of medicine, and my mother's Lutheran church attendance were minor problems in the entire affair. To be sure, the next few years would be characterized by major, unexpected, and seemingly unmanageable events.

Several months after my father's health crisis commenced, the erecting of a cancer center at the RLS hospital began. Prior to its completion, patients were treated at a particular section of the hospital. Although this area was relatively small in its appearance, I found the medical staff to be very professional, sensitive, and approachable. I recall one occasion when a party was held for the patients, and their loved ones. My mother, who was an avid baker, prepared a sweet bread for the function. Other food and drinks at the event included cakes, tarts, pies, punch, sodas, baked macaroni and cheese, peas and rice, stew chicken, stuffing, potato salad, maubi, and an assortment of fruit and vegetable salads. To be sure, it was a joyous affair for one and all. Several months after my father's chemotherapy started, construction of the Charlotte Kimmelman Cancer Center was finalized. It is an attractive, state of the art medical facility. For the next few years, my father would continue his weekly treks to the center to treat his illness. As always, he was accompanied by my mother, who, although she hated to be in the hospital, was committed to be by my father's side throughout his ailment.

Using an umbrella or a cane, because she was plagued by arthritis in her leg, my mother journeyed faithfully to the hospital with him. Additionally, it was very common for her to walk with a transistor radio to the cancer center to listen to music and news on the various local radio stations. Sometimes the time spent at the hospital went quickly; however, there were many days when my parents waited for several hours before the chemo was administered. Moreover, there were numerous occasions when they had to wait a very long time before my father was vaccinated with the drugs to build up his white blood cells. To be sure, as the years passed by, these monotonous hospital visits took a serious physical and mental toll on my parents. After a number of years, although my mother continued to go with my father to the hospital for his chemotherapy, during those occasions when my father was feeling well enough, she would stay at home. Clearly, there were many days when the medicine made him sick, while he was in the hospital, and/or when he was at home. It was at these times when he needed transportation to and from the cancer center. Of course, this affected him psychologically because, as noted earlier, my father had always been an independent person who would drive and do other things for himself. Because my mother never learned how to drive, my parents hired taxis or had family and friends to provide transportation. Mrs. Andrews, a neighbor and family friend, was one such person who drove my parents to and from the Kimmelman Center. After using at most three different taxi drivers, my father settled on one man, Mr. Donovan. Mr. Donovan became my father's personal taxi driver for medical purposes, grocery shopping, and other daily activities.

Looking back, I would say that my father experienced better days than periods that were miserable. On occasions when his health and mindset were not low, he was given a break from the chemotherapy. The range of these breaks lasted from one to three weeks. The summer of 2006 was a time when he was up and about the house, as well as St. Thomas. My oldest brother and his family traveled from Florida to be with my parents at the time. Fortunately, my father was feeling well enough to drive them around the island and spend quality time with them in public areas and at home. Meanwhile, my mother cooked meals, such as conch, fish, and chicken and rice for everyone. They all took pictures at parks and visited other family and friends. Certainly, my mother was happy to get a break and relax from her stressful schedule. However, one day while touring St. Thomas, my father began to feel a little woozy, and my brother drove for the rest of the day. I can clearly recall my eldest sibling telling me, at the time, "Derick, we are blessed. Daddy is so fortunate to be with us talking and driving around. I can tell you that I've met some individuals stricken with cancer who are bed ridden. They can't help themselves. Thank God daddy can move around on his own." Yes, it was a blessing to have my father, given his circumstances, in such good spirits and of sound mind.

Shortly after my father's surgery, I returned to Baltimore, Maryland and continued my graduate studies and employment at Morgan State University (MSU). From August 2002 to August 2006, I was a graduate assistant in the graduate history department. After my graduate assistantship was completed, I was hired as a lecturer in the history department, beginning in the fall 2006 semester. Because of this academic arrangement, starting in December 2005, as I previously mentioned, during each school break I was fortunate enough to travel to St. Thomas and visit my family. To be sure my classmates and colleagues were very supportive of me during my father's battle with cancer. Well wishes, prayers, and, ultimately, financial gifts from my co-workers made a significant impact. Over the years, some students also showered me with kind words and presents to help me deal with my father's health crisis. Additionally, associates of Mt. Calvary African Methodist Episcopal church in Towson, Maryland, where my wife has been a very active member since 2008, were compassionate during the entire ordeal. In the same manner, my wife's co-workers were also caring and helpful during the period.

Because I was working on my PhD dissertation at the time that my father became ill, each time that I went to St. Thomas, beginning in December 2005, I was able to do formal and informal research. Whatever time was spared, I read literature and held conversations on matters related to my school project. For instance, every time that my father was being treated with chemo, I examined articles and books from the library. Similarly, during these waiting sessions, I held conversations with other family members and friends who were also waiting for their loved ones to complete their therapy. On some occasions, I was able to schedule interviews and use the data in my research project. A common occurrence was for individuals to pass through the waiting rooms of the cancer center with carts filled with novels, candies, and magazines. Each time that I was given the opportunity, I collected books by authors such as Dan Brown, Tom Clancy, and Richard North Patterson. Although I knew that I did not have the time to read the texts, because I was busy researching and writing my dissertation, I made it a priority to gather as much books as possible with the intention of reading them sometime in the future.

All of 2006 and the first 1/3 of 2007 would be basically the same with regards to my father's health. Those months were marked by rounds of chemotherapy, good days, lousy days, bad news, and pleasant news. Numerous times, my father's oncologist gave him a positive report that included information that the cancer cells were shrinking. As a result of such developments, the physician would cease the treatment for a few days. Thereafter, my father would return to his domestic chores, social engagements, and other regular activities.

My father's doctor was a very interesting individual. A retiree from the mainland United States, at a quick glance, he looked like his age ranged from 90 to 100 years old. Very soft spoken and extremely not talkative, the physician rarely, if ever, gave complete answers to questions. If my mother or anyone else interrogated him further, he would repeat the same answer, provide a vague response, or not answer at all. To be sure, my mother was not a fan of him. More so, my oldest brother did not like him one bit. The issue was not the physician's competency. On the contrary, the problem was his poor communication skills and the lack of data that he provided. On one occasion, my brother became so infuriated with the doctor that he stormed out of the office, rather than losing his temper and assaulting the medical practitioner. In my mother's case, there came a point, during my father's treatment, that she stopped going to the office. While she continued to accompany my father to the cancer center, she refused to enter the doctor's office, whenever he was consulting with my father.

As noted previously, my father's health fluctuated. One time, his health was improving, and he was in good spirits. Then, his medical report would be the exact opposite: more chemo was needed to slow down the spread of the cancer cells, and injections were required to replenish the loss of his healthy cells from the chemo treatment. Next, in March of 2007, my mother called me and said that my father was scheduled to have an emergency surgery in Puerto Rico, and she would like me to come home for it. The oncologist at Schneider hospital informed my parents that the tumor had metastasized to my father's liver. Thereafter, the physician suggested the medical procedure to remove the malignant growth. The surgeon was a highly qualified physician who had made Puerto Rican history when he became the first person on the island to successfully perform a certain type of surgery. To be sure, the oncology operator's background gave me and my family one less thing to worry about with the surgery. After getting the message from my mother, without giving it a second thought, I quickly packed, purchased a ticket, and made plans to travel to Puerto Rico. Prior to leaving Baltimore, I had to arrange for someone to proctor the third quiz for my classes at Morgan State University. Due to the closeness of the History Department family, I did not have any problem securing someone to administer the quiz. However, when I was in Puerto Rico, I missed the oral dissertation defense of one of my classmates. While this was unfortunate, certainly, it was not the end of the world for me because of my father's urgent operation.

Once I had reached the island and had collected my luggage from the airport, I hired a taxi and immediately went to the hospital. Following a few minutes of being lost in the building, I finally found my older brother and my mother in the waiting room. My oldest brother had not made the trip to Puerto Rico. However, he kept in constant communication with me and my mother about our father's status. When my mother saw me, she was so thrilled and giddy. She started to update me on my father's status and what we were to expect following the operation. My brother gave me his usual calm and unexcitable welcome, but I knew that he was also happy that I was at the hospital. The waiting room was filled with patients' relatives and friends anxiously waiting word on their loved ones. After a relatively long wait, a hospital attendee wheeled my father out of the operating room. Prior to the worker transporting him to the recovery room, my mother, my brother, and I were given an opportunity to spend a few seconds with my father in the hallway. The three of us scrutinized him, looking to see if he would react in any way. Unexpectedly, there was none. Still heavily sedated and in pain, my father just laid there on the stretcher. Although he displayed no verbal or physical actions, we were happy that the surgery was successful; that he was still alive.

The next step for my father was the recovery room. Here, for the next few hours, he twitched now and then; however, he spent most of the time sleeping. Subsequently, he came to, he was placed on a liquid diet, and he began communicating with us verbally. Around this time, a nurse gave him a plastic tube with a ball inside of it. The worker instructed my father to blow in the tube frequently, so that the ball could reach the end of the tube. The attendant explained that, by blowing into the tube, my father would strengthen his lungs, and this would help to expedite the recovery process. A fighter, my father-at every opportunity that he was given-would blow air into the tube and push the ball to the end of the plastic pipe. To be sure, his recovery was progressing slowly but surely. Eventually, my father was assigned to another room in the hospital to continue his recuperation. Although this room was a larger one, it still felt cramped with the four of us, for the next couple days, having a monotonous daily life style. This included watching the same programs on tv; helping my father to bathe, dress, eat, and comforting him. While it was not the most comfortable way of life, the four of us had a chance to bond and share a few jokes by reminiscing on old times. For instance, we watched cartoons, which I hadn't seen in a number of years, such as "The Pink Panther." These shows brought back wonderful memories for me and everyone else. Meanwhile, because of our circumstances, my mother and my brother were forced to watch the tv drama, "24." Prior to our stay in the hospital, none of them were fans of the series. However, because there was one tv, limited channels, and-most importantly-the fact that I was a huge fan of "24," the circumstances guaranteed that everyone was going to watch the show, which aired daily. For the rest of the season and for the next subsequent ones, my mother and my brother either watched "24," or they inquired about it.

Next, we made arraignments to stay in a hotel in Puerto Rico, where my father continued his rest and recuperation. To be sure, the bonding continued and included the frequent trips my brother and I made to the Laundromat and to restaurants to purchase breakfast, lunch, and dinner. One morning, I answered a knock on the hotel door. There, to everyone's surprise, stood my wife! I knew that she was going to travel on that particular day to St. Croix, in order to attend her father's 80th birthday party. However, I had no idea that she would stop at the hotel and spend a few hours with us before she left for St. Croix. Around this time, a few of my father's family members and friends stopped by the hotel to visit him. My wife's unexpected appearance and the other visitors certainly amplified my father's spirits. Prior to returning to St. Thomas, my father had an appointment to see his doctor for a post-surgery check up. The medical report was excellent. The physician, a pioneer and well-known surgeon on Puerto Rico, explained that, if it was up to him, my father would not need any more chemotherapy. However, he emphasized that, since he was not the primary care doctor, and he was not there when my father was diagnosed with cancer, he will not make the final decision on whether or not the chemotherapy would continue. Instead, he stressed that the oncologist in St. Thomas would make the ultimate decision. One of the questions that we asked the doctor was if my father would be able to attend a Caribbean cruise that summer. Another question was whether or not my father was restricted to certain foods. In his response, the surgeon stated, "Oh sure! He can attend the cruise. I see no reason why he cannot. Go ahead and enjoy yourself! His diet, listen, you can eat anything that you want: fish, steak, chicken, pork, anything. You do not have to limit yourself. Based on the results of the operation, I think it is fine for you to go on the trip, and it is okay for you to eat as you please." Of course, everyone, especially my father, welcomed this news.

Two days after our consultation with my father's surgeon, my parents and my brother returned to St. Thomas. As for me, I flew back to Baltimore, Maryland, where I continued writing my PhD dissertation and teaching. As in the past, my supervisor and my co-workers were very supportive during these challenging times. What about my classroom duties? Well, during my absence, I was scheduled to give my mid-term exams. After I created a mental list of classmates and co-workers, who could substitute for me, I asked one of the former. Immediately, my colleague empathized with me and agreed to proctor the mid-term exam. Additionally, Carol-Ann's fellow church members continued their prayers for my immediate and extended families. To be sure, the spiritual and emotional encouragement, which I received from my friends, was a tremendous help. Furthermore, during my stay in Puerto Rico, as noted earlier, one of my classmate's defended his PhD dissertation. Prior to departing for the Caribbean, I had already made plans to attend the event, and I was excited to see my cohort's presentation. Although I would have loved to be in the audience for the defense, it was worthwhile for me to be with my family in Puerto Rico. Certainly, my presence improved my father's morale, and I was able to spend valuable time with my brother and my mother.

Meanwhile, my father did attend the family reunion cruise later that summer, and he patronized his regular diet. For awhile, it seemed like life for my family was getting back to "normal." Then, during a health checkup with the St. Thomas oncologist, to the total dismay of all, the doctor told my father that the cancerous tumors had reappeared, and chemotherapy would have to be resumed very shortly. As expected, my father took the news quietly, with a straight face, and with a positive attitude. On the other hand, my mother-who was naturally filled with emotions-took the news very hard. In public, and sometimes behind closed doors, she would cry and lament repeatedly because of the suffering my father would have to experience. Thereafter, the treatment to kill the cancerous cells continued for the next two years. As before, there were times when the tumors dwindled to such a low level that the physician would give my father a break for 1-2 weeks. However, for most of this period, it was the same old weekly routine: chemo and nutrient booster shots, chemo and nutrient booster shots, chemo and nutrient booster shots. Good days and bad days, good days and bad days, good days, and bad days. One terrible episode took place when the doctor gave my father a new type of medication to control the growth of the cancerous cells. As a result of the new drugs, my father could not keep anything down. I remember my mother calling me on the phone, crying and lamenting: "Derick! Derick! Your father has a new medicine, and all he is doing is vomiting, vomiting, vomiting. He vomit so much in the hospital, and he is vomiting a lot at home." Soon thereafter, the oncologist stopped giving my father the novel drugs. Although the unsettled stomach and queasiness ceased, the cycle of good days and bad days persisted.

During one of the pleasant periods, mid-May 2009, my father was given a break for a few days from the chemotherapy because the tumors had decreased. During these periods, it was very common for him to gain a little weight; his face beamed; and he did his regular chores inside and outside of the house. Sometimes, he even sprinted up and down the stairs adjacent to our house and in the general public. With his spirits high, the feelings of his family and friends, who lived in St. Thomas as well as those of us who lived on the mainland United States, were also enhanced. This was an especially happy time for me because I was scheduled to graduate from Morgan State University on May 16, 2009 with a PhD in History. Two months earlier, on March 4, 2009, I successfully defended my dissertation. Accordingly, once the oncologist had given my father the go-ahead to travel, my parents immediately made arrangements to fly to Baltimore, in order to attend my graduation. Ever since 2005, when my father was initially diagnosed with cancer; underwent his first surgery; and began chemotherapy; I often wondered whether or not he would be able to attend the commencement exercise. By the grace and mercy of God, he was well enough to be present at the promotional ceremony.

Once it was settled that my parents were going to come to Maryland, my wife and I began making arrangements for their arrival. We also started to plan a graduation social gathering. Although, at the outset, I was reluctant to have any form of celebration, eventually, I changed my mind and began to wholeheartedly support the notion. They arrived on Thursday the 14th May and left on Monday the 18th. On the day of their arrival, my wife remained at work for a job function, and one of her co-workers and I went to the BWI Airport to greet my parents. Thereafter, we drove them straight to the hotel, where they had reservations. The following day, at 9am, I attended graduation practice for soon-to-be graduates. Next, my wife, along with my parents, picked me up from campus, and we spent the rest of the day shopping for the party, and my mother and father bought gifts for our loved ones in St. Thomas. Then, spontaneously, we drove to Washington, D.C., where we toured the U.S. National Mall. To be sure, my parents were very excited, especially my mother. Although my father enjoyed being a tourist in the nation's capital, he was more concerned about the chilly weather! I can clearly recall seeing him running to and from the car, in order to get out of the cold air. We concluded the day by purchasing a meal at a seafood restaurant: crab cakes, baked potatoes, and corn. The next day, Morgan State University's 133d commencement exercise was held. It was a very emotional day for me and others. On the one hand, I was very happy to be at the conclusion of my graduate studies, following seven painstaking and challenging academic years. On the other hand, my heart became heavy each time I looked in the audience and saw my parents, my wife, and my other relatives and friends who attended the commencement program. In addition to my parents travelling from St. Thomas to Baltimore for the graduation, other family members and friends, who attended the event, journeyed from Virginia, New Jersey, and New York. To everyone's delight, I sat in the first row of students, and my family and friends were sitting in the front row of chairs in the bleachers. Their seat location was to my immediate right, so, throughout the entire program, I constantly and non-verbally communicated with them. Subsequently, one of my cousins told me that, when she arrived at her seat, my mother was sitting and crying. I never asked my mother why she was crying. However, given the circumstances-including the uncertainty of my father's health-it is reasonable to believe that her tears were those of joy.

Because many colleges and universities held their graduation day on the same day as Morgan's, and a large number of people planned to have public celebrations after the promotional event, it was very difficult for Carol-Ann and I to reserve a business establishment for the post-commencement festivity. After contacting several restaurants, assembly halls, and other enterprises and finding no vacancies, we decided to ask a friend, who is also from St. Thomas and an employee of Morgan, if she would host the merrymaking occasion. Our acquaintance granted our request, and the event was held at her home. What a wonderful bash it turned out to be! There was plenty of food, music, drinks, camaraderie, jokes, and picture taking. Some of my wife's co-workers also joined us in the celebration. I distinctly recall my mother, who suffered with pains in her foot and leg, dancing numerous calypso songs and singing. For instance, when the hit song-*Big Girls Rule*-began blasting over the stereo, my mother had a ball on the dance floor, as she did all the body movements that accompanied the tune. Another partygoer, who clearly stands out in my mind, was one of my wife's colleagues-someone who was a native of Alabama. Although she was born and reared in the United States, her performance on the dance floor to rhythm of the calypso music would have convinced anyone, who witnessed her dancing, that she was born in the Caribbean.

The day following the graduation, my parents, my wife, and I went to one of my wife's co-worker's house for dinner. Other individuals were also present at the feast. Similar to the promotional festivity, the ceremonial feast was a great time of sharing and socialization. This was not the first time that my parents had met the host and hostess. Approximately five years earlier, my wife's co-worker and her husband met my parents in St. Thomas. The co-worker was in St. Thomas to participate in a health conference. Following the symposium, my parents gave them a tour of the island. To be sure, it was the beginning a short, but worthwhile, friendship. The following morning, my wife and I prepared my parents' breakfast, and then we drove them to the airport. While their stay in Baltimore was a short one, it was certainly a happy and worrisome free time for everyone.

Not long after my parents returned to St. Thomas, my father resumed his chemotherapy. By the early fall of 2009, my mother had stopped accompanying him to the Schneider hospital because it became too difficult for her to step up into the hired taxi cab. For the last few years, the arthritis in her foot and leg caused much pain, and whenever she climbed into the vehicle, it resulted in a tremendous amount of hurt and discomfort. Additionally, as noted previously, she could no longer tolerate the oncologist's quiet and non-explanatory demeanor. Because the physician was so introverted, my mother often declared, "Listen, if I ever get sick! If I ever get cancer, I do not want my doctor to be your father's own. I want my oncologist to be another person!" She never stopped there. She always pointed out the specific individual who she said was her choice. Because of her preferential doctor's friendliness, his smile, and his overall appearance, my mother made it known to everyone that this doctor was her first choice, in the event that she too became ill. My mother's eventual reluctance to accompany my father to the hospital was further exacerbated due to the fact that, whenever the doctor asked my father how he was feeling, if he was experiencing any problems, and so forth, my father would always respond that he was well, there were no problems, etc. Even if he had been suffering with joint and body pains, diarrhea, vomiting, and/or other ailments, the truthful response was never completely disclosed. Thereafter, the oncologist would make a few notes in a log, remind my father of the next medical appointment's date, and wish him a good day. This repetitious pattern infuriated my mother so much that she abruptly stopped going with my father to the hospital. If she did go, because she was able to bear the pain of getting into the taxi, she would not go with my father into the physician's office for the consultation. As expected, the trips to the Schneider hospital took a heavy emotional and mental toll on my mother as well. Although it was very rare for my father to overtly be in agony and distress, the fact that the treatment area was known for hosting a large number of patients-many of whom my mother knew-her emotional state was deeply and negatively impacted.

In August of 2010, my family suffered a huge blow, when my cousin, who lived in New Jersey, and who had been fighting cancer for the previous seven years, passed away. Because she had been diagnosed with the disease two years earlier than my father, when it was announced that my father had it, my cousin counseled and advised him about the ailment. She provided him with suggestions on how he could mentally and physically cope with the sickness. She alerted him about what to expect following rounds of chemotherapy and surgery. For certain, my father and my cousin formed their own little informal support group. At this time, it was often very common for my mother to do her own research on how to combat the disease, and it was also a regular practice for her to encourage me to seek out remedies online about how to fight cancer. To say that she was obsessed and consumed with the causes and cures of cancer would be an understatement. To be sure, it consumed her mind and her spare time completely! Even so, the sharing of heath tips, diet plans, and other forms of addressing the illness were normally circulated among my parents, my cousin, and me. Consequently, with the passing of my cousin, everyone suffered a tremendous psychological loss.

A few days before my cousin died, my wife and I went to a New York hospital to visit her. She had been admitted to the medical facility, and her prognosis was not good. Although she could not communicate with anyone in the room, when we arrived, it was meaningful spending time with my dying cousin and other family members and friends. Soon after we made a quick stopover, we drove back to Baltimore. Later, we got the disappointing news of her passing. Once my parents were informed of the death, my mother expressed interest in attending the funeral. On the contrary, my father articulated his desire to remain in St. Thomas. I am certain that he did not fly to the states because he felt that his presence at the funeral would have been too much mental and emotional pain for him to endure. I am convinced that this was the case because, about two years earlier, my mother informed me that he had stopped attending funerals, in general, and, especially, if the person was afflicted with cancer. Meanwhile, my mother faced a major dilemma: she certainly wanted to be present at her niece's memorial service and interment; however, she wholeheartedly did not want to travel without her spouse. Even though my maternal grandmother, my two aunts, and other relatives and friends planned to travel from St. Thomas to New Jersey for the going away mass, my mother was still reluctant to make the journey without my father. For the next couple days, many people, myself included, wondered what would be the solution. Then, one Sunday morning, while I was at church, I received a telephone call from my eldest brother. When I realized who the caller was, I immediately became alarmed because I thought that something had happened to my father. After I gathered my nerves and calmed down a little, I stepped outside and answered the phone. My oldest sibling was calling to tell me that our brother, who resided in St .Thomas, had agreed to accompany our mother to the states for the funeral. Whew! We all breathed a sigh of relief and planned our next step.

My mother, her sister, and my brother stayed with my cousin and her family in Virginia, and then they drove New Jersey for the funeral service. Along the way, they made a stop at a casino and dining establishment in Delaware. On many occasions, my cousin told me that they had a great time, particularly my mother, in Delaware. Although the trip was for a somber reason, they amused themselves tremendously at the gaming and eating business. In the interim, my wife, my cousin-who was a student at Johns Hopkins University-and I drove from Maryland to New Jersey. When we reached the church's parking lot, my oldest brother, his wife, and their newborn son were just arriving to park too, having driven from Florida. Subsequently, my grandmother, an aunt, and a cousin, who had all flown from the U.S. Virgin Islands, showed up to pay their respects. There were several other relatives and friends, some who I had not seen for many years, present at the sad home going service. The following day, a sacrament and interment of my beloved cousin were held. Ever since the death and burial, in the early nine-teen nineties, of one of my most dearly loved senior cousins in St, Thomas, I have been a total wreck at funerals. The Catholic mass of my cousin in New Jersey was no exception. Once I started to weep uncontrollably, Carol-Ann, thank God, was there to comfort me. At the same time, my mother was just as emotionally distraught. For example, after the service ended and everyone was leaving the church, my mother turned to me and yelled, "Derick, do you think this is how your father will be!?! Huh? Do you think this is how his funeral will be?" Dumbfounded and speechless, I could not utter a word in response to my mother's questions. Instead,

I just did my best to regain my composure and console her during this time of bereavement.

Next, a large number of mourners went to a hall where the repast was held. Although we gathered for a very solemn occasion, the event was merry, and it truly felt like a family reunion. There were at least four generations of relatives at the affair. My grandmother represented the oldest age bracket, followed by my mother and her siblings. Even though the first two generations were all confined to wheel chairs and/or had other ailments, they all mingled, smiled for the group pictures, and unrestrainedly ate and drank from the offerings spread out on the buffet table. My first cousins and I comprised the third age range, and their off spring made up the fourth generation. To be sure, it was the first time so many family members and friends were together since my deceased's cousin's wedding in New York in June of 1987. Leaving the repast was a depressing time for everyone; however, the next day, a smaller number of us assembled at my dearly departed relative's home for another reception. Meanwhile, my nephew, his sister, and my brother's wife looked after my father in St. Thomas. During the time that my mother and my brother were in the states for the funeral, my father did not have to undergo any rounds of chemotherapy, and he remained in good health.

In early December of 2010, I travelled to St. Thomas, during Morgan State University's Christmas break, and returned to Baltimore in mid-January of 2011. While I was in St. Thomas, I escorted my father to the hospital for his chemotherapy treatments and consultations with his oncologist. Certainly, my time home gave my mother a physical and mental break from being my father's primary care provider. Once I came back to the states and resumed teaching for the spring 2011 semester, I continued the routine of juggling my personal life and doing as much as possible to maintain my parents' sanity and health. In the meantime, my parents continued their regimen: my father went through his cycles of medical attention, and my mother carried on her task of taking care of him and herself. During these episodes, it seemed that every time my father's health improved, he gained weight, and he seemed to be winning the battle against the *nightmare* known as cancer, his fortunes began to take a beating. For instance, in June of 2011, my father and I watched the NBA Finals between the Miami Heat and the Dallas Mavericks. The nights that we spent together watching and discussing the games were wonderful and momentous occasions. However, in February 2011, which was six months after my cousin's death and burial, the destiny of my family took a turn for the worse. We were the recipients of such horrible and unimaginable news! The reality that my father was being treated for stage four cancer for the last six years was terrible. To say that the new information we got was catastrophic would be an understatement.

Part 2

The Continuance

Chapter 2

My Mother's Diagnosis and Treatment

Accordingly, one day in February 2011, I was in our Baltimore apartment working on my dissertation, cooking, cleaning, and enjoying my day off from teaching classes at Morgan. Since I would not be at school that day, my plan was to do my regular 30-40 minute exercise walk in the neighborhood later in the evening. While taking a break from my writing project, I answered a telephone call. It was my eldest brother who was calling from Florida. After we exchanged greetings, he asked me what I was doing. Then, he took a few deep breaths, sighed, and said, "Derick, mammy has cancer." Upon hearing those four words, I immediately went into a minor state of shock, and my entire body began to tense up. I was silent, so he repeated himself. When I had finally mustered enough nerves and senses to talk, I could only repeat his declaration but with total disbelief, puzzlement, and inquiry. "How did you find out? How did mammy find out? When was she diagnosed? How is she doing? How is daddy doing? How bad is it?" These were some of the questions that I asked my brother. Because he had newly found out about the news, he did not know too much information. As a result, the rest of my inquiries would have to remain unanswered for the near future.

As time went by, I learned more and more details about the cancer, for instance, what type it was, where it was located, when it appeared, and the status of it. I subsequently learned that, from as early as November 2010, my mother began seeing spots of blood in her panty after urinating and wiping. Although I never discussed this particular matter with her, I knew she was traumatized, shocked, and worried about the development. I am certain that she knew it was a possible sign of cancer, the *BIG C* as she and I often referred to it, initially, when my father was diagnosed with it, and the ramifications of the illness. I am sure that, because of her nerve wrecking fear and uncertainty, it is the main reason why she did not tell anyone about what she observed. For the balance of the year, it is my understanding that the spots of blood appeared irregularly. Then, my mother confided in her long time friend and former co-worker what she had been seeing off and on, for the last several weeks, whenever she went to the use the bathroom. Around the same time, my mother also told her sister, a retired nurse who was living in New York, and a few other people. The acquaintance, who I noted earlier is also my godmother, provided support and assurance to my mother. She also encouraged my mother to travel to nearby Puerto Rico and get a medical examination and opinion of the development. However, my mother was very reluctant to make the journey. Instead, she decided to visit a well known St. Thomas gynecologist who was a schoolmate.

Accompanied by her buddy, my mother hesitatingly underwent the tests. She was very unenthusiastic to take the health inspections because she loathed visiting the doctor. Later on, I would learn that my mother let many years pass by before she took any women related medical exams. Nevertheless, due to the circumstances, she went to the OB/GYN's office and underwent tests that she should have been taking regularly. Although she unwillingly had her blood pressure and other basic vitals tested frequently, she usually bypassed overall health checks, especially the investigations for women. Upon getting the results, the physician assured my mother that everything was okay; the spots in her underwear were not anything to worry about; and they would stop appearing shortly. Well, he was partially correct because she no longer saw the remnants for a short while. However, they subsequently began to appear again sporadically. To say that the OB/GYN misdiagnosed my mother would be to make a serious underestimation. This claim is true because, as I would learn later, there were previous verbal accusations of malpractice made against the doctor. For instance, around the time of my father's diagnosis, I clearly remember being told by my mother that one of our cousins, who was later diagnosed with cancer and died, had noticed spots of blood in her underwear after urinating and wiping. The relative went to the same doctor, who my mother would also see about her issue, and the OB/GYN basically gave our cousin the same prognosis as he did my mother. Nevertheless, after observing the traces of blood again, my mother tried earnestly to get in touch with the doctor, but he was never available for one reason or another. Eventually, my godmother was able to give him my mother's message, and his response was an unprofessional, coldhearted, and uncaring one. As it was later revealed to me, the physician told my godmother, (paraphrase) "Well, what do you want me to do? What does she want from me? Why is she calling me repeatedly!?! I told her already what to expect?!"

As noted before, even before visiting the St. Thomas OB/GYN office, my godmother had pleaded with my mother to travel to Puerto Rico and get a full health check up there. It was very common for my godmother to go overseas, whether it was to Puerto Rico or the U.S. mainland, to get her medical exams. Of course, my mother never went with her because, as stated earlier, she despised getting her checkups. However, after the St. Thomas doctor responded to my godmother the way that he did, my mother agreed to fly to Puerto Rico and get a Dilation and Curettage (D & C). Accompanied by her comrade, my mother went to the doctor and underwent the procedure. Later on, my godmother told me that the physician had no difficulty performing the exam. On the contrary, the OB/GYN in St. Thomas expressed that he had a major challenge conducting the test in its entirety because of the excess of tissue in my mother. Upon hearing of the St. Thomas physician's trouble, his Puerto Rican counterpart uttered total dismay and confusion as to why a licensed doctor could not perform a D & C. I recall my godmother telling me, "Listen, Derick, that first doctor your mother saw in Puerto did not have any problems with the medical procedure. He did everything he had to do right there in his office!"

Following the test, the medical practitioner told my mother and her faithful pal that he found an overabundance of material. He emphasized that he did not like what he had seen, and there was too much tissue in the area. As a result, he instructed them to pay a visit to one of his colleagues on the island. After he made the call to his cohort and provided further information, my mother and my godmother took a taxi to the other Puerto Rican doctor. Upon completion of the examination, he informed them that he would send samples of the tissue to another office for additional testing, and that someone would contact my mother and let her know her next step. Thereafter, my mother and my godmother returned to St. Thomas and waited word from the doctor. As can be expected, it must have been a colossal worrying time for my mother. "Exactly what is wrong with me? Will the doctor find something wrong with me that requires surgery? If I do need an operation, who will take care of Elmo (my father's first name)? Who will take care of my grandson (my brother's son who lives in St. Thomas)? Who will pay the bills? Who will take care of the house?" Although I never discussed these specific topics with her, I am 100% sure that these were some of the many questions that rocked my mother's mind daily: night and day. Thank God my godmother was available to offer words of comfort and other means of support to my mother during this inconvenient time. My other relatives and family friends, who lived in St. Thomas and on the US mainland, also provided gestures of assurance and encouragement. However, my godmother was definitely the person who stepped up to the plate and went out of her way to assist my mother.

In the medical office, my mother, my godmother, and my father-my father was also on the first trip to see the Puerto Rican OB/GYN-waited anxiously to hear the results of the test. Then, the doctor said the words that no one wanted to hear (paraphrase): "Mrs. Hendricks, you have cancer." My godmother told me that there was silence in the room for a while. She said that she could see tears in my father's eyes. Without a doubt, he was terrified because he knew that my mother would not be strong enough to endure the mental and physical pain caused by cancer treatment. Having experienced the agony and discomfort for almost six years, he already understood what the diagnosis meant. Meanwhile, my mother searched the room with her eyes, prayed, and continuously sneaked a peek at my father. Again, it is certain that questions about his welfare crossed her mind, just as questions about her wellbeing crossed his. Unlike my father's diagnosis, my mother had uterus cancer, and we would later learn that it was at stage 2. Consequently, she would have to undergo a full hysterectomy. The surgery was scheduled to take place in Puerto Rico on March 10, 2011. In the meantime, my parents and my godmother returned to St. Thomas. At home, my mother attended church, as usual, where a special prayer session was held for her. Her senior high school class also organized a program to pray for her health and recuperation. To be sure, my mother had a lot of support in the days leading up to her operation. Two days prior to the surgery, my parents and my godmother went to Puerto Rico and made arrangements to stay in a locally owned small guest house.

Even though my mother notified me that she saw the OB/GYN in St. Thomas, and she had to take a D & C in Puerto Rico, she never disclosed to me that she had been stricken with cancer. As noted previously, it was my brother, who lives in Florida, who alerted me about her illness. Once I learned of the development, my mother and I spoke, and she asked me if I would be able to come to Puerto Rico for the operation. From my standpoint, the question was not, if I would be present for the procedure. On the contrary, the question was on what day I would arrive on the island. After assuring her that I would be there, I immediately made plans for the trip. It was de ja vu all over again. It felt like as if I was reliving a nightmare again because in the summer of 2005, I had to make an emergency trip to St. Thomas for my father's surgery to remove cancerous tumors in his colon. Then, two years later in March of 2007, I made an urgent trip to Puerto for my father's second operation to take out cancerous growth. Now, in March of 2011, I had to schedule another emergency flight to Puerto Rico for my mother's operation. Moreover, like in 2005 and 2007, I had to make arrangements for someone to cover my absence from work: my graduate assistantship and my lecture position at Morgan State University, respectively. Amazingly, since I had to make the spontaneous trip, I missed another dissertation defense, which was one that I really looked forward to attending. Despite the displeasures, due my absence, I knew that it was essential for me to be in Puerto Rico for my mother's benefit. While I would have liked to remain in Baltimore for the defense, etc., there is nothing that would have taken priority over my mother's care. Like my father, she was always there for me and, therefore, it was my duty, as her son, to be at her side in her time of need.

To say that my morning itinerary to Puerto Rico was nerve shattering and filled with uncertainty would be a huge understatement. Endless thoughts of "why my mother?" and "what is next for my parents?" raced through my mind as my wife drove me to the BWI airport. Although I reached the terminal early enough to catch my departure flight, it seemed like an entire day went by before I actually boarded the plane. The fact that I am afraid of flying and hate it made the circumstances of the excursion even more deplorable. As noted earlier, each time I travel, I am able to attain some sort of relaxation because of two things: I watch the movie shown on the plane, and I read a book during the flight. While the tactic does not calm me down entirely, it diminishes the dissatisfaction significantly. This was also the case on my flight to Puerto Rico. Prior to my arrival, my mother had made arraignments with the owner of the local guest house to pick me up from the airport. After I gathered my luggage, it took a few minutes before my driver arrived. Accompanied by her adolescent son, who was still in his school uniform and who looked like he was in the second grade, we all headed in the direction of the guest house. Immediately, I could tell that the entrepreneur was a hard worker who did not let the fact that she was a single parent prevent her from accomplishing her life's goals. For instance, before we reached our destination, she made three stops that were somehow related to one of her many business ventures. Although I was anxious to see my mother, I did not complain about the stopovers because the business owner's son kept me entertained with his antics. Even though, during our short car ride, the youngster spoke only Spanish, his clowning around allowed me to relax and stop worrying for a little while about my mother's anticipated surgery.

When the automobile pulled into the parking space of the manor, I quickly got my luggage from the car trunk and followed our host to the entrance gate. There, I noticed two individuals standing. One was my oldest brother's former girl friend. Just as she had traveled to St. Thomas in 2005 for my father's operation, she had made the trip to Puerto Rico for my mother's surgery. I could not identify who the person was besides her. Initially, I wondered if it was her son who I had met several years before. Erroneously, I said to myself, "Wow! He has gotten big!" Then, I later learned that it was not her son, but that the individual was her acquaintance. At first, he seemed slightly anti-social and unfriendly. However, he eventually changed his demeanor and appeared to be just another relative or friend of the family. After I greeted the both of them, I went upstairs on the second floor to be with my parents. The first person, who I acknowledged on the second level, was my mother's good friend, standing outside of her quarters. Her husband, who was also on the island for medical treatment, was in their room, watching television. As noted earlier, my god mother and my mother were very devoted to each other, so it was no surprise to me when I observed the former at the guest house. Next, I walked down the hall to the room, where my parents were staying, and I met my parents. It was an ambivalent feeling. On the one hand, I was most definitely happy to be with my parents. On the other hand, I was sad to be there because my mother would have to undergo a serious medical procedure. Absent were my two older brothers. My oldest sibling remained in Florida, and my other brother stayed in St. Thomas.

When my father saw me, he was grinning from ear to ear, and he was asking me one hundred questions per minute! I didn't mind. He was just happy to see me because he knew that, with me being there in Puerto Rico, my mother's nervousness would ease just a little. I know that he was also glad that I was there because my presence would give him less to worry about and simultaneously fewer tasks to complete. I subsequently learned from my god mother that my father was supposed to remain in St. Thomas, so that he could get medical treatment. However, he was determined to be in Puerto Rico, as long as he could, throughout my mother's ordeal. Additionally, he refused to get chemotherapy while away from St. Thomas. Although he knew that, given the state of his health, there was not much that he could do in Puerto Rico, he still wanted to be with my mother. While others and I would have liked for him not to miss his doctor's appointment, we could not fault him for his actions. I sincerely believe that, if he had remained in St. Thomas, it would have done more harm to him psychologically and, consequently, physically. Meanwhile, as my mother expressed her delight of seeing me, from the very beginning, I could tell that she was nervous about her health status. You see, my mother did not worry only about herself, but she was also concerned about other family members and friends, more so, than we were about ourselves. After we all had re-connected with each other, next, we established our plan for the next day. Basically, we were all supposed to get up early enough to arrive at the hospital for pre-surgery check in at 7am. Without any hesitation, our hostess agreed to drive us to the hospital. While the guest house owner left the medical complex and attended to her personal affairs, the rest of us were committed to staying at the hospital as long as possible.

Even though we arrived to the surgical section of the hospital very early, the waiting room was overflowing with the family and friends of many patients. One of my mother's sisters, who lived in St. Thomas, met us there and remained with us for support. The first step was to register the ill person's name and other personal identification information. As the time passed, every one tried to keep a positive attitude and make a few jokes now and then. Meanwhile, one by one, a staff worker would call patients and take them to certain rooms inside the surgical ward. Because we were all so nervous, especially my mother, it seemed that the waiting period would never end. Finally, when my mother's name was called, I got a hesitant feeling. On the one hand, I was happy and relieved because the day was progressing. On the other hand, I was saddened that the next stage was the actual surgery. The medical staff said that one or more persons could accompany my mother to the surgical ward to help her undress, safeguard her personal belongings, etc. My father expressed his desire not to go with her, so I did. To be sure, he could not be criticized because it was a very emotional time for everyone. Once my mother and I got to the designated section, a nurse came into the cubicle and gave us instructions on what was our next step. Although I made a sincere effort to be calm and to appear confident, deep inside, I was very nervous because of the ongoing situation. Certainly, my mother was a lot more anxious and jumpy than I was. I recall that, when my mother was removing her clothes and prepping herself, she received a telephone call from the mother of my nephew who resides in St. Thomas. Because it was very common for this lady to tease my mother, once my mother recognized the voice of the person who had called her, she immediately attempted to end the phone conversation. She said, "Yes. Yes! Okay, I have to go. Bye. Bye!" Next, my mother and I waited for a few more minutes for a nurse to come for her and to take her farther into the operating area. We didn't talk much, while she rested on the bed and apprehensively waited for someone to come for her. Then, a nurse came and transported her to the surgical room. Thereafter, I returned to the section where my father, god mother, and the loved ones of other patients passed the time and worried. .

Next, we all waited and waited and waited and waited. In the meantime, I called family and friends and received calls from a number of individuals who requested updates on the status of my mother. At times, I became overwhelmed with the calls and having to repeat the same thing over and over: "We're still waiting. Daddy is holding up okay. When I learn anything about mammy, I will let you know." Then, after a few hours, the surgeon came to the waiting room and called those of us who would like to get an update. To be sure, we were all nervous about the report. Nonetheless, my father, my aunt, and I went forward to meet with the doctor. Even though my father encouraged my god mother to accompany us, she remained seated and did not consult with the surgeon at that time. In a nutshell, the physician said that he removed as much of the tumors as possible. He emphasized that, because of my mother's previous medical procedures (including three caesarean sections), she had some stuff in the immediate area, where the operation took place, so it was not possible to get everything out of my mother that needed to be detached. Subsequently, when my mother was admitted, he explained to us in her hospital room that my mother's cancer was at stage two, and she would have to undergo chemotherapy. Specifically, he suggested that she take three rounds of chemo, take a break, and then take another three rounds. Thereafter, he said that she should not have to take anymore of the treatment. Without a doubt, the information that the surgeon conveyed was optimistic. Certainly, it could have been much worse. He alerted us that my mother was in a recovery room and, very shortly, thereafter, we went and visited her.

Whew! What a relief. While the road ahead towards recovery was going to be a major challenge, this critical part of the process was over. Next, it was my job to call relatives and friends and notify them of the doctor's details. As I expected, many questions were directed at me that I had no answer for. However, I was able to maintain my composure and sanity. After her stay in the hospital and the doctors determined that she was well enough to be discharged, we prepared to return to the guest house. By this time, my eldest brother's ex-girlfriend and her companion had returned to their home in Florida. For the whole of the first day that my mother was recuperating at the guest house, she was in uninterrupted pain and discomfort. Although my god mother, my father, and I tried our best to ease her suffering, we were unsuccessful in this task. To be sure, prior to leaving the hospital, the physicians explained to us that it was expected that my mother would experience soreness for the next few days. However, the hurt that was afflicting her was totally unanticipated. At one time, my mother began crying and saying, "Something is wrong! Something is wrong! I don't feel right." I honestly thought that she was being delirious and was simply overacting to the fact that she was another statistic, i.e., a cancer patient who was recovering from a major medical operation. Soon thereafter, while she was urinating, my mother started to say that her underwear felt damp, and it was unusual because she knew she had not peed on herself. While helping her get off of the toilet bowl, we realized that there was a small amount of blood in her panty. It was pure panic, thereafter. As I recall it, my mother seemed to be in a daze, totally confused, and scared. After we all discussed the possibilities of what caused the blood, we decided that my mother urgently needed to go to the emergency room (ER). Once we notified the owner of the dwelling what was going on, she called the hospital for an ambulance to get my mother and transport her to the ER. Next, we collected our personal belongings, the guest house owner gave us a blanket for my mother to use at the hospital, and I made a few calls to family and friends, notifying them of the unforeseen developments.

Soon, thereafter, we were ready to leave for the hospital. However, in the midst of all the chaos, I realized that I could not find my cell phone! Where could it be? I had just used it to make some calls, so it was incredible that I had lost my phone. After the ambulance had arrived, it took a few minutes to maneuver my mother out of the room and into the ambulance for this unexpected journey. My father and I rode in the ambulance with my mother, and the guest house owner drove my god mother to the hospital. Thereafter, the proprietor returned to guest house. Luckily, someone later found my phone, and I was able to continue making and receiving calls. My mother was taken to the ER before the rest of us, and we met her inside the establishment. What a night! My mother was one of numerous other patients who waited on hospital beds along the walls of the ER. She was fortunate enough to have a bed to lie down on, while she waited. Some people were standing, and some were sitting. Additionally, the building was freezing. Minute after minute and hour and hour passed from late evening to midnight to early the next morning before my mother was attended to. Meanwhile, my father was trying to be brave, act calm, and remain awake. Thank God my god mother was there with us to keep him company and to observe him. Then, without warning, my mother began vomiting a dark, thick, liquid. To be sure, she vomited a vast amount of the substance, for what seemed to be a long period of time, all over herself and on the floor.

More uncertainty. More anxiety. More apprehension. Finally, she stopped, and we all worked to clean her up. Finally, a doctor examined her briefly and gave us his diagnosis. In layman's terms, (paraphrase) the physician said that one scenario was that my mother would have to be operated on again because she was not stitched up properly. As one can imagine, the information amplified the stress and worries that we were all dealing with at the time. I recall calling my brother's ex-girlfriend and telling her what the doctor said. She immediately cautioned me to make certain that the prognosis was correct because sometimes they are not. She also told me that a friend of hers recently had to be operated on again because, like the doctor's projection, her acquaintance was not closed up correctly. Another point the physician made was that my mother's intestines were knotted, for lack of a better word and, as a result, there was a blockage. Shortly thereafter, another physician asked me if my mother had been stooling and passing gas, after she had left the hospital, initially. When I told him yes, he totally dismissed the blockage theory and, subsequently, he said to disregard the idea that my mother would need surgery again. Interestingly, the first medical practitioner, who briefly examined my mother when she had vomited and told me the blockage notion, vanished from the area. I did not see him again, and I did not care to be in his presence again, since he had made such an erroneous assessment of my mother's condition.

Fortunately, my mother did not have to undergo another surgery, and the doctor's prognosis was wrong. However, he did tell us that a tube would have to be inserted in my mother's nose, down her throat, and into her stomach to pump out the bile like stuff that she had vomited. I accompanied my mother into the examination room, and my father and my god mother remained outside in the hallway. As the doctor made the insertion, he instructed my mother that she should breathe and swallow as she normally does. Although I knew she was petrified with the physician's words, and what he was about to do, she slowly complied with his directives. Meanwhile, I turned my head in the opposite direction because I absolutely could not stand to see what was happening to my mother. Every now and then, she would make a gurgling sound, and the doctor would attempt to calm her and reassure her. We remained in the room for the next few hours, while my godmother and my father stayed in the hallway and soon after took a taxi back to the lodging.

After my mother underwent several hours of the procedure, she was assigned a bed in the emergency room. I remained by her side for the entire night. For me, it was a time marked by hunger, freezing temperatures, uncertainty, discomfort, and an unpleasant sleep. To be sure, I will never forget that night. I remember assisting the technician who tended to my mother and was very nurturing to her. Because of his demeanor, he became one of the many hospital practitioners who my mother liked.

Due to the bitter temperature, I gave my mother my blanket, so that she could be warmer. I was aware of the fact that she never liked to be cold. I tossed and turned in my chair, trying to fall asleep; I trembled repeatedly because of how chilly it was; and I took a few walks in the ER to clear my mind. At one point, I remember getting snacks and a drink from the vending machine. Meanwhile, my mother lay prostrate in the bed and complained to me regularly that she was so cold. To be sure, that night was sad and rough for the both of us, especially my mother.

Finally, my mother was admitted for the second time and transferred to a room on one of the floors. Once again, I made calls to family and friends and gave them updates on my mother's status. In due course, my father and my god mother came to the hospital. When they arrived, the tube was still inserted in my mother, and she wore tightly fitted leg support stockings. Every now and then, one of the nurses would come into the room and measure the amount of liquid that been pumped out of my mother. The tube was subsequently removed; however, my mother did not verbally communicate with anyone until a few hours later. It was such a pleasure to see her open her eyes and to hear her voice. She spent the next few days in the hospital room recuperating. Because I was on spring break from my job, I was able to spend most of the time with her, my father, and my god parent in Puerto Rico. Additionally, my god mother's husband, who was also getting a medical procedure done at the medical facility, visited my mother during her hospital stay.

The next few days were monotonous and uncertain, even though my mother's *physical* health began to improve on a daily basis, in my opinion. I emphasize *physical* because, from my standpoint, during her stay in the hospital, my mother's mental state

began to deteriorate. I am not trained in psychology or any other behavioral science;

however, from what I observed, during the hospital stay, each and every day, my

mother's mental condition declined. For example, she regularly had extreme mood

swings. These patterns ranged from laughing to crying. They also went from talking to

keeping silent, while just staring into space. Additionally, I observed on several

occasions when she would have a good appetite and other times when she would

simply refuse to eat, even though her visitors pleaded with her that it was very important

for her to eat, so that she can fully recuperate. I also witnessed my mother screaming

and yelling with such terror each time one of the nurses drew her blood. During one

such bout, the health worker did not have a difficult time finding one of my mother's

small veins and, as a result, she was very cooperative and satisfied with the procedure.

Soon thereafter, my mother asked the medical practitioner to explain why it was not

challenging to remove the blood sample. Upon finding out from the nurse that a

particular needle, known as a butterfly, was used, my mother demanded from the

nurses that this is the only type of instrument that should be used on her in the future,

whenever they wanted to take her blood. "Butterfly! Butterfly! I want the butterfly

needle. Give me the butterfly needle." Well, for the next two sessions, my mother had

no problem with the butterfly needle being used on her. However, by the third occasion,

it was back to the norm: she yelled, cried, screamed, twisted, tossed in the bed, and did

all sorts of other body and verbal actions to try to ease the pain. As I reflect on those

unpleasant episodes with my mother cringing and being an emotional wreck, I am convinced that my mother suffered some type of mental relapse during her hospital stay.

As a result of my observations, at my first opportunity, I expressed my feelings about my mother's mental state to her surgeon. Although I felt I was clear and logical with what I had been witnessing, surprisingly, the physician totally disregarded what I was saying and completely blew me aside. He told me that her roller coaster behavior was expected, and I had nothing to worry about. To be sure, I was upset and disappointed with the doctor because of his response. Meanwhile, my mother continued to enjoy the attention that this particular doctor gave her. The mere sight of him or mention of his name brightened my mother's face and boosted her attitude. While there were two additional persons, who operated on my mother and visited her regularly, she was head over heels with her primary surgeon. On one occasion, she proudly and willingly took a photo with him. Due to her appreciation of the main doctor, I did not challenge him when he rejected my thoughts on my mother having a nervous breakdown, and I reluctantly accepted his explanation.

The days that my mother spent at the hospital were sometimes pleasant, but, for the most part, they were monotonous, stressful, and tiring. Each night, with the exception of one, I slept uncomfortably on a cot in the room. My father and my god mother returned to the guest house, in the evening, and they came back to visit my mother early the next morning. The usual routine was that, prior to them leaving the hospital, I would ask my father to bring my underwear and clothes to the hospital when he returned the following morning. To be sure, my mother liked my company at night, and I enjoyed the time that I was able to spend with her. Although the both of us did have some happy memorable times, after my father and my god mother left the facility, there were a few unpleasant times. For example, the chief surgeon instructed my mother that it was very important for her to walk the halls regularly, so that she would not get a blood clot in her legs. Initially, my mother followed her favorite caretaker's directives, but shortly thereafter, she began decreasing the amount of time that she walked. Whenever I reminded her of what the doctor had said, she would get upset with me and state, "Listen! I have finished walking already. Leave me alone!" Even if I had accompanied her on a walk in the hallway at 5am, after she had finished urinating, she would often declare, "Okay, that's enough walking for me for today. No more!" At first, I would be angry with her attitude, but then, I began to accept it and no longer pushed her to do her essential walks.

During these nights, I helped my mother out of the bed, walked with her to the restroom, and made sure that her diapers were attached properly. Certainly, many of these episodes were marked with much hilarity and laughter. At least for me, they were. For example, one night while I was on the couch sleeping, I felt an object hit me. After I had awakened, I noticed my mother watching me with a perplexed look on her face and heard her shouting, "Lord, Derick. Derick! Do you know how long I have been trying to wake you? Why do you sleep so hard!?! I want to use the bathroom. Come and help me. I was throwing all sorts of things at you. Didn't you feel anything hit you? I threw the box of tissue, and I hit you with a sheet. I threw a blanket at you. Lord, man. Geez!" Although my mother was frustrated at me, I found the incident to be very funny. After she was finished with the bathroom, she asked me to help her fix her diaper. I did.

She said, "Thanks. Now, come and walk with me in the hall, so that I can get my exercise. But, before we go, I want you to make sure that the diaper is fixed correctly. Is it? I don't want to be walking and it falls off." I assured her that it was taped on properly, and it would not come off during our walk. Well, as soon as we left the room and began to make our way down the corridor, to my mother's alarm and to my surprise, the diapers began falling off! While my mother protested and complained about what was happening, I hurriedly re-attached the clothing. To be sure, my mother took the matter very seriously, whereas, I found the incident to be hysterical.

As noted previously, the few days that we spent at the medical facility were sometimes repetitive and dull. Usually, I would buy myself breakfast early every morning. Then, shortly after I had finished eating, my father and my god mother showed up to the hospital to visit my mother. We all chatted, made jokes, and scrutinized the nurses and doctors as they examined my mother. On many occasions, I volunteered to buy my father and my god mother lunch and/or dinner. There were times when they accepted, and there days when they did not. Because my father was a very thrifty person, he usually refused my offer and wanted me to buy meals with his money and not my own savings. One time, he shouted, "Derick. Use my money to buy lunch. You don't have any money. You need your money. You are using your money to buy food, drinks, linen for your mother, and all sorts of other things. Here Here! Use mine! You broke. You broke!" It was common for me to laugh at my father's offer to use his money and not mine; however, on this particular day, I was very upset. In my frustration, I yelled, "Daddy. I have my own money. I can buy lunch and other things. It's okay. Look, look!" I was in such an emotional wreck that I almost threw my cash in the air as an act of disapproval of my father's words. Once my godmother noticed what was going on, she intervened and calmed me and my father down. The few times that my godmother's husband visited my mother, he also took part in our reminiscing, story telling, and other socializing. Similarly, my mother's sister, who was in the waiting room on the day of the surgery, also visited my mother during these times.

Unsurprisingly, some nurses were more memorable than others. For instance, there was a Puerto Rican nurse who my mother became emotionally attached to. My mother's strong affection was for two reasons: 1. The nurse was very nice and 2. My mother said that the nurse resembled my maternal grandmother. One day, we learned that my mother would relocate from one hospital room to another. When my mother learned of this development, she instructed me to search for the nurse and to tell her about the room change. Unfortunately, I did not find the nurse, and I had no recollection of her name. To say that she was an angel, who was sent to look after my mother to nurture her and to help her recuperate, is not fantasy. Up to this day, I believe that the nurse was one of my mother's guardian angels, and I do not make any efforts to explain the nurse's sudden presence and then disappearance. Similarly, my mother and I observed that my father was very fond of another nurse who was a black American woman. Each time she came into the room, my father's face would lighten up, and he would begin speaking in Spanish. Sometimes, he would talk English in a Yankee accent. While my mother verbally expressed hostility towards his frolics, I found my father's behavior and my mother's reaction to it as totally amusing. To be sure, even though the days that my mother spent hospitalized were mostly filled with the same daily routines, the times were still marked by laughter and much needed camaraderie.

Meanwhile, I meticulously took notes whenever the medical practitioners examined my mother, and I was certain to ask them questions about my mother's health. Consequently, I also developed a bond with the doctors and nurses. Several times, they commented to my mother that I was a faithful son, one who was dedicated to the improvement of her health status. Along these lines, they frequently told my mother that she was fortunate to have such a "loving son" because they knew of many cases where individuals were hospitalized and neither family nor friends would visit them. My response was simply to smile and to tell them thanks for their kind words. My mother also usually smiled, nodded her head in agreement, and would say silently, "Yes, he is. Thank you Jesus." Without a doubt, my note takings were beneficial because, by writing them, everyone could follow the progress/status of my mother's health. For example, we all monitored her blood pressure, body temperature, and other vital signs on a regular basis.

Certainly, the stress and worries of witnessing my mother in the hospital had a physical and mental impact on everyone who visited her. Unsurprisingly, my mother also suffered from the state of affairs. For example, one day when she had no appetite, my father kept urging her to eat her food. He continuously uttered, "Eat Eleanor. Eat! You need to eat. Do you remember when I was not eating, and you kept telling me that I need to eat my food? You need to eat Eleanor, so you can get better." Although his intentions were noble, my mother would not accept them. At one point, she shouted, "Why don't you just shut your mouth and leave me alone!?!" Thereafter, she uttered something to the effect that he was happy to see her in her present state. This was such a horrible time for me, my father, and everyone else who heard the anger, pain, and sadness in my mother's voice. Immediately, my father became quiet and retreated into his own private little shell. I did my best to avoid eye contact with him, but this was almost impossible due to the room's small size. For certain, it would not be the last outburst from my mother to those around her.

After I spent a few days and nights, right next to my mother's bedside, consulting with the doctors, shopping in the hospital stores for daily necessities, I was exhausted emotionally and physically. My depressing state was noticeable to everyone, who visited my mother, so my father encouraged me to take a break and spend the night away from the hospital. Over and over, he kept asking me, "Aren't you tired? Aren't you sleepy? You need to sleep. Stay in the guest house tonight and get some rest." Initially, I resisted his advice, but, ultimately, I relented because I desperately needed to clear my mind and to take a time out. Although my father was the leading advocate for me to spend one night away from the hospital, he was hesitant to have me leave the building because he was convinced that I would not know how to unlock and lock the gate to the visitors' dwelling. However, after demonstrating to me several times what I needed to do, in order to access the holiday home and after my god mother assured him that I would be okay, he conceded. Not surprisingly, I had no problems whatsoever with the gate, and I had a wonderful sleep that night.

Once I returned to the medical facility the next day, I quickly resumed the duties and the daily routine of assisting my mother. For example, on multiple occasions, she continued to suffer the pain of injections and having to undergo exams of her stomach, back, and other body parts. There was at least one instance when she had to submit herself to an ultrasound. Additionally, I can clearly recall one time when, after we had

newly returned to the hospital room, following an x-ray examination, a staff member

came to us, announcing to me and my mother that he was instructed to take her down

stairs for another x-ray procedure. To be sure, I was surprised by the worker's

declaration, but I kept my feelings to myself. However, my mother expressed disgust

and protested loudly. She screamed, "What!?! Where? When? Again!?! I just came

back from doing an x-ray. No, no, no. I said no! I am not going back for another one!

Not me." Like many other times, this incident left me with a feeling of two minds. On

the one hand, I thought that the entire episode was funny because of my mother's

boisterous theatrical behavior. At the same time, however, I was unhappy because of

the mental anguish and uncertainty that I knew she was suffering. As in the past, while

my mother was being examined, I was responsible for calling my cousin in Virginia and

other people and provide them with an update of the most recent medical test.

Meanwhile, my brother, who was residing in Florida, made his regular phone calls to

find out how our mother was doing.

I cannot stop emphasizing that my job at Morgan State University was

convenient and understanding of my family crises. In most other firms, I believe the

situation would have been largely different. However, with Morgan, I was allowed to

use my breaks, as well as when school was in session, to travel home and to take care

of my parents and other family issues. Interestingly, when my parents had their

surgeries in Puerto Rico and, during other occasions, the period coincided with summer,

Christmas, or some other type of school vacations. As noted earlier, in the event that

classes were in session, I never had a problem identifying someone (whether it was my wife or a colleague) to substitute for me each time classes resumed. The knowledge that my employer would not penalize me for my absences surely reduced my psychological pain in these times of emergency and uncertainty.

After we had received word that a hospital discharge date was set for my mother, everyone was elated and overjoyed, even though we all knew that many challenges were in the future recovery period. In the midst of our excitement, one day, one of the doctors came in the room and glumly told my mother that something unexpected happened, and the day of departure would be delayed. Naturally, we were all immediately saddened, especially, my mother. Then, the same doctor calmly told my mother, "Mrs. Hendricks, I must tell you, I am only joking. You will be released from the hospital as planned!" My mother, like everyone else in the room, was speechless. Although this particular physician was known to us for being a joker, this most recent comedic antic caught us all off guard. To be sure, we all laughed loudly and resumed our activities, preparing for the day that my mother would leave the medical facility.

For example, we were informed that certain discharge notices, my mother's St. Thomas mailing address, etc. had to be filled out. Under normal circumstances, my father would have willingly left the room and completed all the necessary forms. However, because he had bypassed his chemo treatment, in order to be with my mother during her operation, he was getting weaker and weaker every day. As a result, I accompanied him to the various offices and filled out the forms with him. I wretchedly recall the day when a staff member asked my mother to complete a document related to her discharge. For some reason(s), she was very uncooperative and reluctant to sign the papers. At one point, she shouted, "Why don't you all just send me to St. Thomas and let me die! What is it that you all want me to sign? Is it my death papers!?!" I sincerely believe that my mother was so mentally and physically stressed out, at this time, that she really did not understand what exactly the hospital worker was simply requesting. To be sure, this was a tremendously nerve wrecking time for me. It truly was. Nevertheless, after coaxing by those of us in the hospital room, especially my god mother, my mother finally signed the release forms.

Shortly thereafter, my mother was released from the hospital. Prior to her discharge, as noted previously, she was informed that she would have to undergo three rounds of chemotherapy, take a break from it, and then, if she was up to it, she would have three additional sessions of chemo. Immediately, based on my father's reaction to the medicine, I knew that she would not be able to tolerate the drugs. My mother despised any type of vaccination, blood test, and all other medical exams. Because a willing and brave mindset was mandatory for patients to triumph over cancer, we all knew that my mother's recovery would be a slow and an uphill battle. For instance, as previously noted, she would cry frequently, while she was in the hospital, and she would sometimes refuse to eat. On one such day, I lost my temper and shouted, "Mammy, you have to eat. You have to stop crying! If you can't take these hospital injections now, how in the world are you going to deal with chemotherapy?" To be sure, I was frustrated with my mother, while simultaneously, I was angry with myself because I had allowed my feelings to explode uncontrollably. Nonetheless, life continued, and we took up residence again in the guest house. A couple days after the discharge, I flew back to Baltimore, Maryland. The hours leading up to my departure from the guest house were depressing and heartbreaking for everyone. Then, when it was finally time for me to leave the building and head for the airport, my mother started to cry louder and louder. Even though my father and my god mother tried to calm her down and to reassure her that I would travel back to St. Thomas ASAP, my mother continued to moan and weep and cry. As I exited the room and the bed room, I could still hear her groans and cries of anguish. Meanwhile, my cousin in Virginia and other persons made suggestions that my brother, who lived in St. Thomas, should accompany my parents from Puerto Rico to St. Thomas because my mother and father were both weak and in poor health. Despite the ideas, my brother remained in St. Thomas and made arrangements for my parents' arrival. Thank God my god mother was available and kind enough to escort them to the airport and to St. Thomas.

Because I was drained mentally, during my stay in Puerto Rico, one would think that I would be at ease, well rested, and relaxed in Baltimore. However, nothing could be further from the truth. While on the U.S. mainland, my emotions were unresolved: On the one hand, I wanted to be in St. Thomas with my parents. Yet, I wanted to be in Baltimore with my wife. As a result of this dilemma, I constantly wondered about the welfare of my parents. Questions, such as, "Were they in pain? Were they comfortable? Were they feeling alone and abandoned? Were they hungry? And were they taking their medications?" raced through my mind twenty-four hours a day. Even though I knew that my parents were being assisted with their daily activities by my god mother and my brother, I still pondered on the interests of my father and my mother. Furthermore, although I was able to teach my classes, smile, attend church, go to the movies, and do other normal daily activities, I was hurting badly inside. Night time was the worst! Every other night, I experienced a nightmare. Generally speaking, they were the same. They were not scary dreams filled with terror. On the contrary, my nocturnal thoughts, basically, were that I was still in Puerto at the hospital with my mother. During these nights, whenever my wife got out of bed, I would wake up and say, "Mammy, mammy! Are you okay? Where are you going? Do you need me to help you to the bathroom?" In a soothing voice, my wife would always say, "It is okay, Derick. You are not in Puerto Rico anymore. You are here in Baltimore with me, your wife, Carol-Ann." Sometimes, in the middle of the night, I would stretch my hand towards her, touch her, and refer to her as my mother. My nightmares and other nocturnal horrific episodes were so awful that there were times when I even got out of the bed and attempted to follow my wife out of the room, thinking that she was my mother, who was in the hospital, and needed some type of help. On these occasions, after giving me her reassurance that my parents were fine, and everything was okay, I would return to the bed and fall asleep.

As I implied before, after my mother went into surgery, she was never the same person. Never. This first became clear to me, while I stayed with her in the hospital, and it became evident to everyone else immediately after she returned to St. Thomas. For instance, when I was in Baltimore, my god mother, my brother, and my father often told me over the telephone that my mother spent her days in cycles of crying and being happy. After I returned home in May of 2011, I saw for myself what I had been told about my mother. To describe her behavior, feelings, and attitude as riding on a rollercoaster would be a conservative statement. Based on what I witnessed in St.

Thomas, I sincerely feel that exactly what I told my mother's surgeon-that she had undergone some type of nervous breakdown in the hospital-was confirmed.

Because Morgan has two summer sessions, from 2011 to 2013, I made it a practice to go to St. Thomas for the first summer term and then return to Baltimore to teach the second summer session. Moreover, as previously noted, during these two years, I made sure that I went to St. Thomas for the Christmas, Thanksgiving, and spring breaks. Without a doubt, these two years marked the saddest and most exasperating eras of my life. During my stays in St. Thomas, it was common to observe my mother talking, laughing, and being herself. Then, suddenly and without warning, she would just change her disposition! Thereafter, she would start weeping and basically shut down. No one knew what was going on. We were all puzzled and confused as to why my mother was such an emotional wreck. Feeling helpless and irritated with myself because I was unable to help her, I contacted a psychologist at the Roy Lester Schneider hospital and explained to her my mother's medical history and her current erratic behavior. Following a series of questions, for example, if my mother usually became upset and disoriented once the sun began to set, the psychologist concluded that my mother was suffering from the early stages of dementia. She informed me that, while the illness was not reversible, steps could be taken to slow down dementia's progression. Immediately after our conversation, I began to recall instances involving my mother that were clearly suggestive of an individual who was stricken with the illness. One case in point occurred one late afternoon when my parents were resting on their bed, and I was in the room just to keep them company. Out of the blue, my mother started to say, "Derick, Derick, come and take this thing off of my back." I didn't see anything there, so I told her that she had nothing on her back. I informed her that the only thing on her back was her blouse. Upon hearing this, she got aggravated, began to suck her teeth, and said, "Come on, man! Come take this thing off my back. What is it that is scrawling on it!?!" As far back as I can remember, my mother was drastically afraid of lizards and wood slaves. She was not terrified of insects. However, like small reptiles, she never wanted insects crawling on her body.

A few minutes later, my mother shouted, "Derick, come mop up this water on the floor! Come pick up these papers on the ground!" Without any inspection of the area, I was one hundred percent sure that the floor was dry, and there were no pieces of paper on the ground. I told this to my mother, but she wholeheartedly refused to accept what I was saying. By this time, my father was just as confused as I was. I remember he leaned over to my mother and calmly said, "Eleanor, what are you talking about? There is nothing on the ground. There is nothing on your back. Go back to sleep." I added, "Mammy, these things are in your head. There is nothing on the floor or on your back." Well, my mother went in a rage! She yelled, "Listen, why don't the two of you leave me alone!?! Derick, what you mean by 'it is in my head?' You are not a doctor.'" In reply, my father said, "Eleanor, do you know who you are talking to? This is Derick. It's Derick you are talking to." Again, my mother sucked her teeth in utter annoyance and bellowed, "Yes, he is a doctor, but he is not that kind of doctor!" To say that the entire episode made me sick to my stomach would be an understatement. What was even more demoralizing was that my mother was exhibiting signs of the early stages of dementia, and I did nothing to help her. Although I was unaware of her illness, I still felt guilty because of my actions and inactions.

Another example of my mother showing signs of a mental disability involved me and my brother. Prior to her surgery, my mother took drugs to control her blood pressure. One afternoon, she asked my brother to get her bag, so that she could get her pressure pills. He did. The question was, "Had she already taken the required dosage for the day?" Other questions surrounding the matter were, "Did she still have to take the medication, since she was recovering from surgery? Was she supposed to take the entire prescribed amount?" Even though the doctors in Puerto Rico and the doctors in St. Thomas had previously answered all of the aforementioned inquiries, the three of us were unsure of the correct answers. What a calamity. What a confusion. For the next several minutes, the three of us were going in circles about what should be done, in order to resolve the matter. Even after we all reached a consensus on what we should do, my mother subsequently decided to doubt whether or not we were doing the right thing, and she began to cry. Then, she started to blame me and my brother and accuse us of not understanding her predicament. Viewing this affair in retrospect, I am certain that my mother's behavior was involuntary. She could not help her words and deeds because she was ill and, as noted before, no one knew that she was experiencing the beginning stages of dementia.

Sadly, my mother also forgot how to bathe. I recall, one day in early May of 2011 when I was in St. Thomas, I was in the bathroom, assisting my mother. After she had soaped up the washcloth, she asked me, "What should I do now? Where should I wipe?" This was so dispiriting and depressing for me to witness. Around this same time, my mother refused to have conversations on the telephone with her family and friends. This was totally unlike her because, for many years, she would speak daily on the phone to her contacts about the weather, the latest gossip, health, and other issues. For example, her brother, who lived in Florida, called her every day or vice versa, and they reminisced about their childhood, life in the states, and Virgin Islands news. Then, one day, out of the blue, he called me and asked me, "Derick, what is wrong with Eleanor? What is wrong you with your mother? I called her to talk to see how she is doing today, and she would not talk to me. This is not the first time that she did this." I could not believe what I was hearing because my uncle was known for calling my mother and harassing her by playing pranks on her. Although my mother usually scolded him for his shenanigans, they both would have a good laugh at the jokes. On another occasion, my brother, who lived in Florida, called me with a similar complaint about our mother's unfriendly phone conversations. For years, she called him and others on the U.S. mainland to alert them about pending weather forecasts and other natural and manmade disasters in their areas. Consequently, my mother's response to him, one day, left him so confused and at a loss that he reached out to me to find out what was going on with her. He said that, after he had greeted her and asked her how she was doing, she replied curtly. Then, he asked her about the weather in St. Thomas. Thereafter, she said, (paraphrasing), "There is no weather. There is no weather!" He said that, the next thing he knew, he was speaking to our father. Obviously, she had abruptly given him the phone, so that he could talk to my brother. The new behavior even affected my grandmother. She related to me, one day, that, during a phone conversation, she had asked my mother how she was feeling. Her unexpected response to my grandmother was, "I sick! I sick!" Then, she handed over the phone to my father. I remained in disbelief of these stories, until I visited St. Thomas and noticed them for myself.

Another disturbing example of my mother's unpredictable behavior involved my brother's trip to St. Thomas, shortly after my mother returned there to recuperate. Once my mother was informed that he was coming to check on her and my father, she was filled with high expectations to see him. During normal times, there would be no drama on the day of his appearance in St. Thomas. However, by the time he planned to visit my parents, my mother had already started to show signs of dementia's early phase. Accordingly, on the day of his arrival, a tiny faux pas resulted in a full blown commotion. I subsequently found out from Annette, my cousin, who lived in Virginia, that arrangements were made for my brother, who lived in St. Thomas, to travel to the Cyril E. King airport and to meet our eldest sibling. He went to the airport, as planned, but my brother was not one of the passengers who came off of the plane from Florida. As a result, my brother called our mother and asked her to verify that our sibling was scheduled to travel on a particular airline. When she did, he reported to her that my oldest brother was not on the jet. Furthermore, he told my mother that there were no more scheduled flights to St. Thomas from Florida on that particular airline. Well, according to my cousin, upon hearing that my brother did not disembark off of the airliner, to paraphrase, "all hell broke loose!" Annette relayed to me that my mother called her screaming and crying, saying that my eldest brother was not on the plane. She yelled that he was supposed to be on it, but my brother, who was supposed to pick up the new arrival, called her and said he was not on the aircraft. Apparently, my mother was wailing, fussing uncontrollably, and giving my cousin an earful, clearly expressing her disappointment that her son was not at the airport as planned. We later realized that my mother's actions were unnecessary because there was a mistake in the correct arrival time and/or the name of the airline. Once again, it must be emphasized that, under ordinary circumstances, my mother would not have behaved in this manner, but given that she was uncertain about her health's future and being a victim of a debilitating mind sickness, her words and actions were excusable.

During this episode's mishap, I was still in Baltimore, and individuals, who spent time around my mother, continued to provide me updates on the well-being of my parents. To be sure, the time that my oldest brother spent in St. Thomas was not a pleasurable one for him. For example, he related to me that, one day when he was assisting our mother from one part of the house to the other, she began to wobble, fall backwards, and screamed, "Butch, hold me! Hold me!" Thank God he was walking right behind her, so he was able to catch her as she fell. In my opinion, my mother experienced some type of fainting spell because she was still weak and learning how to walk. Although she did not totally pass out or collapse to the ground, to be sure, it was a scary moment for everyone, especially, my brother. As I mentioned earlier, Butch Cletis, and I grew up in a household where our parents were never truly sick, so it was a psychological shock for me and my siblings when our parents were both diagnosed with cancer and battled to overcome it. Hence, when she had the operation in Puerto Rico, and when she buckled backwards on that particular day into my brother's arms, I knew both incidents traumatized him beyond his imagination, and I sincerely believe they are two of the principal reasons why he only visited my ailing parents twice during the two years that they were both severely incapacitated: 2011-2013.

Following my mother's operation, the surgeons used staples to close her open wound. The physicians informed us that she did not have to return to the hospital to have the surgical pins removed from her lower stomach area. On the contrary, the fasteners would just disintegrate on their own. Moreover, we were advised that, until all of the clips had diminished and disappeared, someone would have to clean and dress the wound, and this person would also have to administer injections to my mother, in order to prevent blood clots. Like my mother, I did not have the willpower to follow the doctor's instructions to treat the cut and to give the vaccinations. Thank God my god mother had the strength of mind and the fortitude to carry out the doctor's directives. Out of pure love, she came to the house and took care of my mother's wound. To be sure, my mother and everyone else truly appreciated the dedication, commitment, and resolve of my godmother to take a leadership role in the recuperation of her beloved friend: my mother. In addition to her nurturing, my godmother also stepped up to the plate in a variety of other areas. For instance, she brought tapioca, cream of wheat, and other hot cereals for my parents' breakfast every day. Those times, when my godmother had already made plans not to be at the house, she fixed an extra amount of cereal for my parents and placed it in the refrigerator for them. It should be noted that, once my mother returned to St. Thomas from Puerto Rico, she refused to enter the kitchen for anything, including, cooking, to wash dishes, and to get food/drink items from the refrigerator. Interestingly, my father also stopped going into the kitchen, shortly thereafter. Neither of them would even get a cup of ice for themselves. Instead, my godmother, Cletis, or I would fetch everything that they needed. Although their behavioral pattern was new and strange to me, I never criticized them for the novel trend. I am sure that others did not find fault in my parents either. In addition to preparing breakfast for my parents, sometimes, my godmother would go to a restaurant and bring lunch for them. During the times that she was unavailable to do this, or for some other reason, Cletis would get their lunch and bring it to the house.

In addition to providing breakfast and lunch for my parents, my godmother also did their laundry. Whenever I traveled to St. Thomas to visit my parents, I would assist her in washing, drying, and folding clothes and other linen. Although these were tedious and stressful days for me, I was still able to find humor in them. For instance, although my godmother would repeatedly tell me and show me how to fold fitted sheets, for the life of me, I would always complete this task incorrectly! Every now and then, I would do it quickly and secretively, but she always caught me in my shenanigans, and we often had a good laugh. The practice of my godmother doing the laundry would continue for a long period, until a misunderstanding with Cletis resulted in her no longer doing the task. Thereafter, he would wash the dirty linen, when I was in Baltimore, and I would take care of it whenever I visited St. Thomas. Meanwhile, my godmother continued to help my parents with their daily regular household tasks. For example, immediately after my parents and my godmother returned to St. Thomas, my father resumed his chemotherapy sessions. By this time, he had already topped driving his car. As a result, my godmother or a taxi would take him to and from the hospital for treatment and wherever else he desired to go. Similarly, my godmother also transported my mother to the hospital for chemo and other places in St. Thomas. I must emphasize that my mother's friend never asked for compensation, favors, or anything else for her services. Everything that she did for my parents and for my family was done simply out of pure love. This, I will never forget.

As I noted earlier, in early May, immediately after I had administered the spring 2011 final exams, graded them, and submitted the scores in Morgan's online grading system, I boarded a jet and headed to St. Thomas, so that I could help my parents recuperate from their illnesses. My plan was to remain on the island for the first summer session of Morgan, and then return to Baltimore in late June/early July, so that I could teach for the second summer session. Without any thought, I followed his regimen for the next two years. During the early summer of 2011, it became clear to me and others that my father was losing more and more weight. Although it was common for his weight to fluctuate, due to the ramifications of chemo, in May of 2011, I noticed that his body mass was decreasing steadily. For example, at one point, the medicine affected his gums, and it became painful for him to eat solid food. After mentioning this development to his primary oncologist at the Schneider hospital, the doctor prescribed a certain medication for my father to take, in order to alleviate the discomfort in his mouth. Although my father did purchase the drugs and took it as directed, he still had a difficult time consuming food. Meanwhile, he got thinner and thinner as the days progressed. A lover of breadsticks, one day, he ate a few pieces of them and stored the rest away, so he could have them for dinner. However, when it was time for him eat the breadsticks, it was just too agonizing for him to complete the task. With much frustration and disappointment, I recall seeing my father throw his hands up in the air, suck his teeth, and grumble that he was not able to eat the breadsticks. To say that it was so heartrending to see him expressing such sadness would be a grave understatement.

Shortly after this incident, my godmother asked him if he was taking the pain relief medicine that he physician had recommended, and he answered affirmatively. Then, she said, "Listen, Elmo, are you sure that you are taking the correct medicine? Let me see the note from the doctor and the medicine bottle." After scanning both items, she said aloud, "But Elmo! Do you know what is wrong? You bought the wrong medicine. This is old. You are not taking the correct medication!" Wow. What an oversight! Right away, she made it her mission to get the correct drugs that the doctor had suggested that my father take to ease the soreness in his mouth. As expected, thereafter, it became easier for him to chew and swallow food because he was now using the correct medication. Unfortunately, in my opinion, my father never regained his weight after this incident. Ever since, I have often wondered whether or not his health would have declined as rapidly as did, if this avoidable error had not taken place.

Furthermore, when I accompanied my father to the bank, the hospital, and other establishments, it became clearer and clearer to me that he was suffering not only physically but also psychologically. As noted earlier, my father was a very independent person. He was a person who never relied on anyone to do things for him, if he was capable of doing them himself. Now, he needed to rely more and more on a walking cane, someone to assist him with completing various activities, and doing other things that, just a few years earlier, he would have done on his own. Although it was very tough on me mentally to witness my father slowing down, we did have a few moments together that were enjoyable and memorable. For example, as I pointed out previously, in June of 2011, my father and I watched the NBA Championship Series between the Miami Heat and the Dallas Mavericks. I do not remember which team he supported, but

I do recall that we had a good time together as we watched the games, discussed the players, and made predictions about who we thought would win the series. Incidentally, to my dismay, the Miami Heat lost the tournament 4-2 to the Dallas Mavericks. Nevertheless, the time that we spent together for the tournament was pleasurable, and it is one of the last enjoyable moments that I spent with my father.

Meanwhile, by the time that I had arrived on the island in May of 2011, even though my mother was still seriously sick, she was well enough to begin her first round of chemotherapy. First, I had to find an oncologist who would attend to her. After doing some research, I was able to locate a doctor at the Schneider hospital to complete the task. He was a perfect fit for my mother because, as I mentioned earlier, beginning in 2005, when my father became a cancer patient, my mother always expressed affection for the same oncologist who I had assigned for her care. Following the Puerto Rican surgeon's instructions, my mother was to undergo three rounds of chemo and then, if she was well enough, to go through three additional bouts of the therapy. Given her distaste of any type of medical procedure and based on how she displayed mood swings following her surgery, we all knew that it would be very difficult for my mother to successfully submit herself to the recommended periods of chemotherapy. However, I did not realize that her fight against the horrible disease would be so timid. Certainly, I am not trivializing the fact that chemotherapy and its side effects are monstrous and almost unbearable. In contrast, I am simply expressing my disbelief in my mother's lack of resilience for the fight of her life.

Although my mother liked her oncologist, her fondness for him was not adequate enough to conquer her fears and apprehension about chemo. As a result, she was an unwilling patient; one who would do almost everything in her power not to cooperate with her primary physician and the nurses. To be sure, my mother was very familiar and friendly with the medical staff because she had interacted with most of them for the previous six years. Nonetheless, her mind, attitude, and behavior were not only embarrassing, but they were wholeheartedly fatalistic. For example, on a regular basis, she did not tell the oncologist and the nursing staff the complete answers to their questions. If she felt that the answer should be yes, her reply was yes. If she believed that the answer should be no, her response was no. Meanwhile, my godmother and I would intervene and attempt to provide the facts and the absolute truth to their inquiries. This only angered and infuriated my mother. On one occasion, she yelled, "Listen, doctor, do not listen to him. He lie! He lie! Derick, get out of here. Get out! I don't want you to come to the hospital with me again because all you are doing is causing trouble!" At the time, I found my mother's actions to be funny, yet disappointing. What is interesting is that, before my mother was diagnosed with cancer, she used to frequently admonish my father for not telling his doctor the entire truth about his health. For instance, one time, he was not feeling well due to a stint with diarrhea, but on the day that he saw his physician and nurses, he told them that he was fine and had no complaints. After hearing this, my mother quietly cried and pleaded with my father to tell the entire truth. Of course, he did not and stuck to his story. Now, ironically, she was doing the exact same thing.

Another example of my mother's uncooperative demeanor took place whenever she had to take her vitals. On one occasion, I witnessed her refuse to stand on the scale to be weighed. While I empathized with her because she was still recuperating from surgery, and her legs were not robust, there was very little evidence that she even tried to board the weighing machine. As a human being and her son, who wanted her to recover from her illness, this lack of will power frustrated and saddened me simultaneously. Then, when my godmother and I offered her encouragement and support, my mother accused us of being against her and not understanding her plight. Of course, this assessment was totally false. By showing such physical and mental weakness, her doctor explained to us that it would be difficult for her to complete the rounds of chemotherapy and, thereafter, regain good health. By this time, my mother's mind was already on a downward freefall. Due to the emerging dementia, it was common for her to lay blame on individuals without any substantiation whatsoever. For instance, one afternoon while my godmother was helping her up the stairs leading to our home's front door, my mother's foot inadvertently grazed against the steps. Thereafter, she began to get upset and later complained that my godmother had deliberately scraped her foot against the steps. Of course, my godmother had not done any such thing. However, in my mother's mind, the act was executed on purpose. Even though my godmother felt deeply hurt by the imaginary accusations, out of love for my mother and my family, she continued to assist us with transportation, meals, essential advice, and other important matters. To be sure, there were days when my mother appeared cheerful and strengthened after getting a dose of chemo (she referred to it as "life water"). But for the most part, the period that she had undergone

chemotherapy was marked by a wanton lack of cooperation and by depression.

That summer, I remained in St. Thomas until the end of June. Thereafter, I

returned to Baltimore to teach summer session II. Accordingly, for the balance of May

and June, I continued to assist my parents to the best of my ability. As in the past, the

time was very tiresome and psychologically nerve-racking. As noted earlier, my mother

had stopped accompanying my father to the hospital, so I escorted him to the grocery,

the hospital, the bank, and other destinations. By this time, he reluctantly walked with a

cane, and it was a real struggle for him to take steps without rocking from side to side.

Since he was always an independent person, he despised having to use the walking

stick. Regardless of the many times that my grandmother and my mother implored him

to use the cane, he hesitated to use it. One day, my grandmother said, "Elmo, why

don't you use the cane? You better walk with it before you fall down!" He brushed off

her urging, but one day, he was walking in the hallway, and I was in the living room or in

the kitchen. All of a sudden, I heard, "bam!" When I rushed to find out what happened,

I saw my father sitting on the ground and with a look of confusion and humiliation on his

face. To be sure, after that incident, my father made it his business to use the walking

stick outdoors. Similarly, my father resisted pleas from my mother to sit down while he

was taking off his pants and putting on a different one. Although he found it difficult to

keep his balance, while he stood and changed his pants, he continually resisted calls for

him to change his traditional method. Like my grandmother, one day, my mother

advised him, "Elmo, Elmo, please sit down when you are going to change your pants,

so that you do not fall down. If you don't sit down, one day you will lose your balance and fall!" Again, because it was common for him, in the past, to stand up and change his clothes, he found it extremely shameful that he was reduced to now having to sit, in order to complete the task.

Moreover, I remember the day when, after he had walked up the steps leading to our front door, he came in the house and literally threw himself on the couch. He was out of breath! This really traumatized me because I knew when my father would run up the steps and not be winded afterwards. When my mother observed how weak and tired he was just from walking up the steps, she started to quietly wail. Another instance, when I noticed her sorrow, due to my father's alteration, occurred on the day that he had taken off his shirt and put on another one. Once he had removed the shirt, his ribs, collar bone, and spine were clearly visible. I quickly noticed it, and I didn't say anything. On the contrary, when my mother saw it, she groaned and cried, "Loooooooorrrrrrrd, Lord have mercy." Upon seeing her reaction, my father just asked her what was wrong and rapidly replaced the shirt. Although he was slowing down a lot; he had lost a significant amount of weight; and it was really challenging for him to walk, my father never wavered about his willingness to get chemotherapy. Certainly, he did not like getting the treatment. However, he remained steadfast in his conviction to get the medicine. One day, while we shared a taxi with some passengers, a strong scent of stool enveloped in the small van. By this time, my father's health was so poor that, sometimes, it became difficult for him to control his bowel movements. Although he did not tell me that he had messed himself, I strongly suspected that it was him because of his body language and the embarrassing look on his face. During another incident, I had to hurriedly escort him from a bank to a public bathroom, so that he could urinate. I willingly held his arm and guided him to the restroom. When we arrived there, a man was standing outside and waiting to use it, also. Then, he turned to us and said, "I can see that he is sick, so you can go ahead in front of me." This act was very humane, and my father and I were very appreciative of the deed.

After it became obvious that my parents needed additional assistance in their day to day lives, I spent a few hours, one afternoon, researching nursing homes and other facilities that could provide that support. I recall that both of my parents were a little hesitant towards my objective. However, my mother was much more open-minded to the idea than my father. To be sure, the representatives of the institutions (public and private) that I contacted were sympathetic to our plight, and they provided valuable information. Meanwhile, I was just shaken emotionally by everything that was happening to my parents and many times I felt as if I was at my wits' end. Thank God my godmother was there to offer me comfort, suggestions, and calm the fears of my parents who were uneasy about me reaching out to nursing homes. I remember her saying, (paraphrase) "Eleanor, Elmo, don't worry. Derick is just looking out for what is best for the both of you. He is looking towards the future, and how you all will be taken care of." In late June/early July of 2011, I returned to Baltimore, so that I could teach summer session II at Morgan State University. When I left St. Thomas, my parents were still living at home. Meanwhile, my godmother, my brother, who lived below my parents in the same house, his wife, my grandmother, and other relatives and friends all supported my parents in one fashion or another.

As in previous years, although I was physically in Baltimore, my mind was in St. Thomas, and I constantly wondered about the welfare of my mother and my father. As a result of this predicament, my nightmares and weight loss continued to afflict me. This challenge was surely made worse because of the reports that I received almost daily from St. Thomas about my parents' wellbeing. Without a doubt, I was caught in an inescapable tight spot. Why? This was the case because, on the one hand, I was eager to get information about what was going on in St. Thomas with my mother and father. On the other hand, I did not want to hear any news about them because, sometimes, the reports were unpleasant. For example, even though it was very important that my mother keep active by walking in doors, I was told frequently that she was reluctant to do this. Similarly, although my father still had a positive mind, regarding his treatment and recovery, I was informed often that he was getting thinner and thinner. Fortunately, my colleague, who is a psychologist at Morgan, and who edited my dissertation chapters, remained in touch and provided counseling to me. Without question, the therapy sessions with him greatly alleviated my troubles.

Then, on the morning of August 3, 2011, I received a telephone call from my brother, who lived in St. Thomas, telling me that our mother had suffered some type of medical emergency. Later, we learned that she had experienced mini strokes in the past, which no one knew about, but on that early August morning, she endured a serious one. What a calamity! What a catastrophe! What horror! In the recent past, my mother had a blood clot in one of her legs and had to receive medical treatment for it. Thereafter, she used a particular equipment to assist her mobility, and it became extremely difficult for her to use the steps. As a result, she would be placed on a special chair, and at least three persons would carry her from the street to the front door of the house and vise versa. Nevertheless, she experienced an urgent situation because of the stroke. Moreover, it is normal, whenever there is some type of crisis, for the first reports to be inaccurate. My mother's case was no exception to this phenomenon. For instance, when she was discharged from the hospital in Puerto Rico and went back to St. Thomas, we were told that her cancerous tumors were restricted only to her uterus. However, that August morning, my brother excitedly told me that the cancer had spread to other places, including her spine and stomach. The family subsequently learned that none of that news was accurate. While she had suffered a stroke and was left paralyzed below the neck, the cancer had not spread to other organs. Even so, Cletis said that, as was usual, he went upstairs early that morning before he went to work, looked at my father and then went in a different room to watch my mother. (At some point in time, in 2011, my father began to sleep in a different bedroom apart from my mother because he could no longer bear her constant crying, screaming, and inability to control her bowel movements). Cletis said that, when he observed our mother in the bed, she was bleeding from her mouth and nose, twisting, turning, and biting her lips. He said that he quickly told our father, who, although he was in a bedroom not too far away, was totally unaware of what had happened to our mother. Next, Cletis, in a panic, ran downstairs and told his wife of the new development. Thereafter, one of them made a call to the Schneider hospital, and an ambulance came for my mother.

As my wife hastily made airline arrangements for my flight from Baltimore to St. Thomas, I continued getting false information about what had happened to my mother and her diagnosis. Although I am sure that none of the news carriers had any bad intentions, the incorrect narratives definitely had a damaging impact on my psyche. In most instances, the gossip reached my ears, but in some cases, it did not. For example, I subsequently learned from one of my childhood friends that, on the morning that my mother was stricken, he was told that she had some type of attack, she had fallen off of the bed, and she was found on the ground several hours later by my brother. As a result of all the confusion, as one can imagine, I was an emotional wreck from the moment that I learned of my mother's sudden illness, until I arrived in St. Thomas a couple days later. Moreover, this dreadful event took place at the worst possible time: the week of final exams. Once again, my loving wife came to the rescue, as she proctored the examination session, graded the tests, and submitted the overall grades. However, for the first time, during the period of my parents' health crisis, there was some controversy due to my absence from my place of work. Simply put, the issue was related to one of my students, who was not present, on the day of the final exam. Although the entire class was given an ample opportunity to take the test earlier than its scheduled date, because of an absence on the day of the test, the aforementioned pupil missed the examination, because, she claimed, she had already made plans to be out of town. She did not alert me of her upcoming trip, so she earned a zero for the final exam. This lowered her final score to a C. She later appealed her score, on the grounds that she had attempted to contact me, while I was in St. Thomas, and the matter was sent to adjudication. My colleagues ultimately ruled against me and in her favor, and I was forced to give her another chance to take the test. I complied, she scored exceptionally well on the test, and her overall grade was changed to a higher score. Looking back, I know that, under different circumstances, I would have handled the situation differently. Thus, I feel that it is because of all the stress that was on my shoulders at the time, it clouded my judgment on how I dealt with the matter. Nevertheless, I do not regret giving her the grade that I originally did, and I am most certainly not sorry that I traveled to St. Thomas so quickly because I knew that my parents needed me by their side during such an uncertain and terrible time.

After taking a few deep breaths and putting on the best relaxed facial expression that I could muster, I departed the airplane in St. Thomas and swiftly gathered my luggage. A few years earlier, without a doubt, my father would have met me there at the airport. However, due to his poor health, he no longer traveled to the air or seaports to greet arriving passengers. Although the car ride to the hospital was a relatively short one, this time, the drive appeared to last much longer than normal. My belief is expected because my mind was overloaded with worry, concern, and apprehension about my mother's status and what I would observe when I met her. After I had signed in at the reception desk, Cletis and I went straight to the Intensive Care Unit where my mother was located. I first noticed she was asleep and resting quietly. Additionally, she was heavily medicated, and tubes were inserted in her mouth and nose. As a result, she did not see nor communicate with me and Cletis. That day, my mother was also visited by my grandmother. One of my cousins, who was at the hospital to see another patient, also checked in on my mother that day. Within three days, she was assigned to a room on a floor of the hospital. During the first couple days there, my father did not come to the hospital. There is no doubt in my mind that, emotionally, it was too much for him to abide, so he stayed away from the medical facility. The other reason, why I believe that he did not come to the hospital at that time was because, physically, he was too weak to make the journey. Well, my feelings were verified, when, shortly thereafter, he did come to the hospital to see my mother. Using a cane, he walked slowly towards the first floor elevator and boarded it. Every step of the way in the lobby, I constantly asked him if he was okay, and if he wanted to me to get a chair for him, so that he could take a break. Unsurprisingly, his response to each one of my inquiries about the chair was "no." Moreover, he regularly denied that he was tired and proclaimed that he did not need to stop. However, when we arrived on the floor of the hospital, where my mother was located, about mid-way to the room, my father leaned against the wall and, almost out of breath, he stated, "Derick, are you going to bring the chair?" What a pitiful sight, and what a miserable condition for me to witness on that day. While my mother was stretched out on a hospital bed and paralyzed from the neck down, my father was leaning up against a hospital wall totally exhausted after walking a few feet. When he was in the room, my mother barely opened her eyes on a couple occasions and, she still was not able to talk with anyone. Instead, she just slept while some of her friends and family members streamed in and out of the room to check on her.

Similar to when my mother was hospitalized in Puerto Rico, one of my tasks was to make telephone calls to her relatives and acquaintances, who resided on the mainland United States, and to give them updates on the status of my mother's health progress, including medical examinations. For instance, on the day that a neurosurgeon performed a lumbar puncture on her, I notified several persons (including my brother who was still in Florida) about the procedure. Similar to our time in Puerto Rico's hospital, I found that the experience of relaying the exact information over and over to several individuals was very tedious and stressful. What was more painful for me was to witness the lumbar puncture exam. In my opinion, the physician handled my mother very roughly when he did this test. For example, at one point, he tossed her on her stomach, and I could see that her face was pinned tightly on the mattress. The scene was so grotesque. I could see that my mother's semi-open eye was rubbing back and forth on the bed. Even though I explained this to the doctor, he impatiently disregarded my complaint and continued steadfastly with the examination. Moreover, as someone who despised needles, I was well aware of the mental and physical trauma that my mother was suffering when this particular test was being performed. Since I am definitely not an enthusiast of injections either, the event was also difficult for me to watch. Because my mother still was not speaking at the time, all she could do was groan and moan during the test. This was one of the many agonizing ordeals that I had to deal with, during this horrible period, when my parents had cancer.

During my mother's stay at the Schneider hospital, this same neurosurgeon told Cletis and me that our mother did not have much longer to leave. In the midst of our expression of sadness and disbelief, he stated, "I do not give your mother long to live. Because of her critical illness, I will give her two weeks before she dies. Two months, the most that I will give her is six months to live." What went through my mind, upon hearing this death sentence that the doctor had just said to us, is much too difficult to reproduce here in words. For sure, I knew I was not ready for her to die; not yet. Some of the numerous things that I thought about were the following: How? Why? Who would tell my father? How would I explain this wretched prognosis to him and other individuals? If it was hard for me to even go over the words in my mind, how could I get them out of my mouth? Eventually, I did have to unwind, bring back myself from wonderland, and explain the doctor's narrative to relatives and friends. As I think back on that conversation with the neurosurgeon that day, it is easy to recognize an absolute difference between his mannerisms and the characteristics of one of the surgeons who performed my father's first cancer operation in 2005. As noted earlier, following that procedure, the surgeon had made clear to us that he would not give a time range for how much longer my father would live. Nonetheless, I quickly realized that my family's future would continue on a challenging and rough path. While I had come to terms with this outlook, undoubtedly, I had no idea of how demanding and taxing it would be.

After my mother was discharged from the hospital in Puerto Rico and returned to St. Thomas, someone suggested to me that I consider placing her in a hospice. Although I had heard this word previously, to be sure, I was still unaware of its meaning. This individual noted that, since my mother was having such a challenging time getting back on the road to full recovery because of her physical, emotional, and behavioral obstacles, hospice care would be the best option. Definitely, I understood that my mother was having a hard time restoring her health and, like everyone else, I wanted what was best for her. As a result, I did a little research on the implication of hospice care. Upon learning its significance and totally aware that, without it, my mother would not have certain resources, I refused to put her in such an institution. Thereafter, I recommitted myself to doing everything in my power, identifying, and using whatever means I could attain to make my mother comfortable and to keep her alive. Nevertheless, after her stroke in August of 2011, the situation became more dire and serious. My mother's physical condition had deteriorated so dramatically that her oncologist instructed me to have her placed in hospice care. This time, there was no debate involved. There was no question; no alternative. He sympathetically and benevolently rationalized his position. One of the reasons that he gave me was that because my mother was now paralyzed and was too weak to continue with chemotherapy, she would need to be assisted 24 hours a day in some type of hospice care facility.

Meanwhile, although my father's weight continued to decline, and his strength diminished daily, he remained resolute about getting chemotherapy. However, when I accompanied him that August for a chemo session, we were both left flabbergasted and dazed by the news that his oncologist had given us. After he had taken my father's vital signs and asked him how he was feeling, the physician, as was his customary modus operandi, read some information from a medical log. Then, he quietly stated: Mr. Hendricks, after many years of surgery and chemotherapy, the drugs no longer have any positive effect on you. Whereas, in the past, the chemo would shrink your tumors, this is no longer happening. Given your age and due to your falling health, I am discontinuing your chemotherapy sessions. On the one hand, the report sounded nice because no more chemo meant that my father would no longer experience the dreadful effects of the medicine. On the other hand, the information was unpleasant because, without the drugs, the cancerous growth would multiply. Next, the doctor said that the cancer had spread to my father's adrenal glands, liver, and other very important organs. Perhaps, the sadness, fear, and uncertainty that the oncologist noticed on our faces were the reasons why he uttered the words that he said next. He stated that there was a new cutting edge experimental drug, which was being used in the mainland United

States, which he said he would try to get for my father. For certain, this new remedy

was no panacea, but, at the moment, it definitely gave some level of relief and

optimism, especially, to my father.

There is a saying: when it rains, it pours. What my family and I were

experiencing was a perfect manifestation of the aforementioned proverb. Imagine,

shortly after my mother was hospitalized and referred to become a hospice care patient,

my father's oncologist had, in essence, "given up" on him and suggested that he also be

placed in the same type of institution as my mother. Unexpectedly, my father tried to

put on his best facial appearance, after hearing the doctor's prognosis. In the office that

day, my father repeatedly pressed the oncologist on the circumstances, availability, and

other matters related to this so-called new experiment. As a matter of fact, for the next

couple days, I recall my father asking me to repeat for him exactly what the physician

had said about the innovative drug. It was very sorrowful for me to see and listen to my

father as he would state, "Derick, what did the doctor say, again? He said there is a

new experimental drug, right? He said he will call and let me know, right? Didn't he say

it might help me?" Sadly, the oncologist never called my father to inform him of these

presumably novice pills. Not once. Eventually, my father stopped talking to me about

what the doctor had said about the trial tablets. As a matter of fact, his disposition had

changed totally. Whereas, in the past my father would willingly go in for chemo, there

came a point when he basically said, "Why should I go back to the doctor? What's the

point? Why am I going to be weighed and checked for other statistics? The doctor said

he will stop giving me the chemo, so I am not going to the hospital anymore." Wow.

Like his physician, clearly, my father had "given up." What a tragic turn of events that my father's mindset had taken. Of course, I never criticized him for his new attitude towards his medical care.

One good thing that took place that August in my father's physician's office was when the doctor provided us with information, regarding hospice care. Aware that my mother's doctor also recommended her to become a home care patient, my father's doctor encouraged me to have my parents simultaneously become a part of the program. In addition to giving me the contact name and phone number of a particular facility, he assured me that he would personally get in touch with the institution and alert its staff that my parents would become two of their newest clients. Moreover, in the midst of all the sorrow, doom, and gloom that I was experiencing, at this time, my mother's cancer doctor told me something that uplifted my spirits to some extent. On this occasion, he pulled me aside and said, "Listen, your father did well. Given his age (in August 2011, my father was 72 years old) and with the type/stage of cancer that he has, he handled himself remarkably. Whereas other individuals, under the same circumstances, would be given a life expectancy of two years, at most, your father is now in his sixth year of battling this illness. Keep this in mind." To be sure, those kind and comforting words gave me a sense of hope and happiness in the middle of this terrible storm that my family and I were confronting. In the meantime, I learned that the type of hospice care that was available for my parents was not in the public sphere. On the contrary, given the state of affairs at the time, they were required to remain at home and would be visited by nurses, doctors, social workers, and a pastor. Immediately, I touched bases with the hospice care firm that the doctor suggested; I made an appointment with the head doctor of the facility; and this physician and the home maker met with me and my father in our home. Following the consultation, including filling out the necessary documents, a date was set for when my mother would receive a hospital bed from the home care facility and the first day of her home care.

Meanwhile, my mother's health was unpredictable. On one occasion, I accompanied her neurologist to a room, where he used a computer monitor to show me the brain injury that my mother had suffered, as a result of her stroke. Later, he told me that, following the recent health scare, she was now a full blown diabetic. However, when I mentioned this subsequently to my mother's oncologist, he told me that my mother was not diabetic, and she was still on the border line. Could you believe this? It was bad enough that I had to hear from the neurologist that my mother had two weeks left to live. Now, her neurologist and oncologist were giving me conflicting diagnoses of her health; absolutely amazing. It seemed as if things were getting worse quicker than they were getting better. Despite the mixed messages and terrible reports, we all remained faithful and prayed for the best. Nevertheless, due to my mother's critical status, my father began making plans for what appeared to be the very near death, funeral, and burial of my mother. Because of all the fears and uncertainties that were prevalent at the time, his vision seemed to be on point. To be sure, no one knew for certain how much longer my mother would live, and he wisely felt that the family needed to be prepared for her anticipated demise. Interestingly, prior to her stroke, because of his rapidly declining physical condition, it was commonly believed by many persons that my father would meet his end first before my mother.

Nevertheless, he began to set his plan in motion. As noted earlier, my mother was a dedicated member of the Frederick Evangelical Lutheran church. However, after my father's cancer diagnosis in 2005, she began to go with him to his home church: New Hernhut Moravian church. Although this was the case, she never renounced her Lutheran membership to become a Moravian. Even so, his plan was to reserve two burial plots in the Moravian church graveyard: one for himself and one for my mother. Unsure whether or not the Moravian pastor would allow my mother to be buried next to him, my father asked my godmother-who was a member of the Moravian church-her thoughts on the matter. He wanted to know if she felt that his plan would be successful. Being the frank and honest person that she is, my godmother told him that she had no idea what the pastor would do, and she suggested that he ask one of his cousins, who was an influential member of the church, to ask the pastor if she would grant my father's request. Accordingly, my cousin posed the question to the pastor, and she agreed to my father's wishes. Whew! Once I learned of the pastor's affirmation, I was overwhelmed with a genuine feeling of ambivalence. On the one hand, I was pleased that both of my parents would be buried side by side, as my father desired. On the other hand, I knew that for this to happen, it meant that both of my parents would have gone on to meet their maker. What a dilemma. What a predicament. What a catch-22.

Next, my god mother drove my father and me to the Moravian churchyard, so that he could select the area of land that he wanted. The cemetery is located on a hill. Consequently, my godmother made sure to travel with a folding chair, so that my father could use it to sit at the bottom of the incline. While the walk from the car to chair's spot was a difficult one for him to make, my father carefully made the short journey. Once he had reached the destination, it did not take too long for him to make his preference known. Following a quick surveillance of the region, he pointed out to my godmother and me exactly where he wanted both vaults to be built. Like many other episodes, for me to witness this spectacle was very tear-jerking and heart breaking. Yet, one positive item from our project in the graveyard that day was knowing that my father's goal was fulfilled. Even though he was extremely weak and could hardly sustain himself, this one gesture that he made, I knew, gave him a sense of satisfaction and pride. After we left the burial ground that day, (or on a different day) my godmother drove us to my parents' bank, so my father and I could sign certain papers. Knowledgeable of the reality that my mother was bed ridden, and he was no longer capable of leaving the house to do financial transactions, we signed documents to have my name appear of the same bank accounts as my parents. This way, when I was in St. Thomas or off island, I could conduct family business in their interests.

The drive to the bank was a very uncomfortable one for my father. At one point, he was actually lying down in the backseat because it was too distressing for him to sit up. The feeling of awkwardness and pain for my father was also present when we were in the banker's office. At one point, the banker and/or I realized that we had made an error with the credentials. When the worker gave us an option of re-doing everything or not modifying it, my father protested filling out new papers because he said that he was tired and just wanted to go home. Seeing him squirming and struggling in the office chair, trying to ease his body aches was so heart trending and pitiful for me. By this time, in addition to him having lost most of his energy and weight, a good amount of his muscles were no longer visible. I recall guiding him to the shower one day. While I was holding him up, as he washed himself, he glanced down on his body, began passing his hand over his chest and grumbled and sucked his teeth in utter frustration, saying, "Look at this. Look at this! What is this? Look at me!" I did my best to comfort him and told him he will be okay. I even tried a little humor by telling him that she should not worry. I assured him that only the both of us were watching his figure, and he was not in a beauty pageant show. To be honest, my father's stature was nothing but skin and bones. I likened his profile to a museum exhibit of prehistoric dinosaurs, the victims of German atrocities that were perpetrated on their southern African colonial subjects, and to images that one might view of Jews who were prisoners in Nazi concentration camps. Initially, when my father walked passed my mother, on his way to and from the restroom, he would call her name and try to get her attention. However, as he became sicker and sicker and more disoriented as the days went by, he would just pass the bed without even acknowledging her.

If there was ever time, when I needed a clone, it was when both of my parents were fighting cancer, especially, when my mother became hospitalized in August of 2011. Back and forth. Up and down. Back and forth. Up and down. Sometimes, I became so totally overwhelmed with trying to get everything in order with my parents that I almost snapped! Primarily, the grace of God and my godmother are the two main reasons why I did not have a physical and a mental break down. Of course, there were other persons who assisted me, besides my godmother, but I can wholeheartedly say that she truly stuck by side and helped me every step of the way. Since taking care of my parents was a new issue really for me, I had to operate by trial and error. Additionally, I learned new things on a daily basis. For example, one day, while my mother was in the Schneider hospital, and I was doing errands for her, an office worker asked me if I was my parents' Power of Attorney (POA). When I told her no, she said that I needed to fill out an application and become one because it would be necessary when I was required to make certain decisions. She explained to me that she had recently become POA for her parents due to their illness. This lady was kind enough to give me a copy of a POA document and advised me that I draft one that was applicable for me. Thereafter, she put me in touch with a Notary Public (NP), who was also a nurse, and she informed me that this Notary Public could assist me in becoming a POA. Next, with the assistance of my wife, who was in Baltimore, I got the essential forms drawn up, the NP stamped them, and I was officially authorized to execute my parents' affairs on their behalf.

Getting my father to sign the documents was easy because he still had the ability to write. However, in my mother's case, she no longer was capable of signing papers because she was paralyzed. As a result, in the presence of the NP and others, I was instructed by the NP to secure the pen in my mother's hand as she marked an "X" on the line where she would normally have written her name. What a poor sight to observe. I would never have dreamed that, one day, I would have to guide my mother's hand and help her to make an "X" on a form because she did not have the physical power to write her own name. Wow. Nonetheless, as the POA for my parents, the physical and mental burden on me was lessened a little. While my mother was out of ICU and on the hospital floor for patients, my oldest brother, Butch, who resided in Florida, came to St. Thomas. Like everyone else, I know it was a shock for him to see our mother in such a state. Once it was decided that our mother would become a patient of home care, and she would get a hospital bed, Butch and I removed our parents' old bed, swept and mopped the bedroom, and made space for the new piece of furniture. Although it was a lot of material that had to be removed, we did it in a timely manner. There were so many decades old cards, letters, papers, and other items that we found in the room. As someone who loves history, I meticulously read everything that I put my hands on. In one funny case, Butch said, "Derick, I don't want us to be here all day. You can't read everything that you find. You can't do that, or we will never finish!" Once again, in the midst of sadness and misery, I was able to find a little laughter.

Prior to my mother's discharge from the Schneider hospital, a heath care worker advised me that her food would have to be pureed. Even though she was still not speaking, my mother was put on a liquid diet while hospitalized. The employee further told me where I could purchase a machine that could mash food into a thick paste. Right away, Cletis and I went to the establishment that was suggested, and we got the purifier and other products that my mother would need. Although my father was also in home care, he was still eating solid food. Additionally, the homemaker, Ms. Day, who my father and I had met earlier, was assigned to work six hours in the house: 8am-2pm from Monday to Friday (M-F). She did not work on Saturdays, for religious purposes; however, I paid her to work for two hours every Sunday from 8am-10am. Subsequently, the hospice reduced her work hours from six to three hours per day: 8am-11am (M-F). Thereafter, I paid her to take care of my parents from 11am-2pm from M-F). Her duties included bathing and feeding my parents. However, my father was strong enough to take showers without her assistance, and he could feed himself. On a regular basis, I would have to call the hospice and put in an order for certain items for my mother, such as pampers, chucks/bed pads, and glucerna energy drinks. On many occasions, the facility did not provide an adequate amount of supplies, or it did not make available the materials that my mother needed, so we would have to purchase certain products ourselves. Meanwhile, my cousin, who lived in Virginia, frequently mailed pampers for my mother. Additional help came from one of my aunts, who lived in St. Thomas, when she sent juices for my mother, and from other relatives and friends-including Butch- who also sent fruits, pampers, and other well-needed items. With the time for me to return to Baltimore rapidly approaching, I did as much running around/running errands as possible in St. Thomas, before I went back to work. Additionally, I made certain to put the medication regimen on the bedroom mirror, so that Cletis or my godmother could give my mother her drugs. Although she was very helpful, there were certain things that Ms. Day did not do, such as giving my parents medication and washing clothes, towels, and other garments. During these times and others, my godmother and Cletis fulfilled the duties. Once my parents were settled in hospice care, Butch returned to Florida, and I flew back to Maryland.

Part 3

The Ending

Chapter 3

My Father's Death and Burial

Shortly after I returned to Baltimore, Morgan State University's fall 2011 semester began and, similar to previous years, I was there in body, but my mind was in St. Thomas. Once I came back to the states, I experienced the usual: nightmares involving my parents' health, counseling by my psychologist colleague on Morgan's campus, factual news and gossip about what was going on with my mother and father, and having to continuously answer inquiries about how my parents were doing, and how I was coping with my family crisis. Then, I went back to St. Thomas to help care for my parents. When I first saw my father, I could tell that he had lost even more weight, since I had last seen him, and I noticed that he needed additional assistance. However, he was well enough to help me select someone who would be a care taker for the night time. While I was still in Baltimore, it became clear to me and everyone else that, even though my brother and his family lived on the first floor of my parents' two story house, my mother and father desperately needed someone who would take care of them during the night. Accordingly, after Ms. Day left the house at 2pm sharp, my godmother usually spent the next three or four hours with my parents, until roughly 5-6pm. Thereafter, Cletis, whose job finished at 4:30pm, would make himself available to my parents. Many times, he had personal business to do, so my parents were left alone for a short period of time. Whenever I came to St. Thomas, I stayed with them 24 hours a day, 7 days a week. However, once I returned to Baltimore, there were periods, especially during the night, when no would watch them. Be that as it may, when my father told me that, once I g to St. Thomas, he advised me to find someone who would work the night shift. Prior to my arrival, there was one lady who made an appointment to meet with my father. However, a few minutes before she arrived at the house, while she was driving and talking to my father on the phone, he told her that her services were no longer needed. I later spoke with the prospective employee, and I was quite embarrassed, after she told me how my father had treated her. I never found out from him exactly why he handled the potential homemaker in the manner that he did. However, I believe that, by this time of his health status, he had even lost confidence in himself to make such a decision.

Nevertheless, my parents still needed a part-time custodian, so I continued to research the matter. One afternoon, Ms. Day gave me the contact information for a lady who was knowledgeable of the home care market in St. Thomas. Ms. Day suggested that I contact this person, and she assured me that this individual would assist me with my project. I followed her instructions, spoke to the person, and she gave me the name and telephone number of a possible worker. Soon thereafter, the prospective laborer, my father, and I met in the living room, and we discussed the job requirements and salary. The interviewee accepted the position, and we all made arrangements for her to begin working the next business day. Amusingly about 2 hours, after the verbal contract was made, the interviewee called me and stated that, given her demanding work hours, she felt that her pay should be higher. Due to the stress and desperation that overwhelmed me at the time, without challenging her plan, I proposed an increase of about $1.25 to my original offer. To my surprise, she quickly accepted the new salary and emphasized that she would be at our house the very next business day. To this day, I strongly believe that the lady, who referred me to the prospective night worker, encouraged the latter to request a higher salary. Even so, the individual, Ms. Night, was not affiliated with any hospice care institution. Quite the opposite, because of her experience as a domestic caretaker, she provided freelance services on St. Thomas. For instance, during the day, from about 8am to 6pm, she did home care work for a nearby elderly couple. In my parents' case, I assigned her to work from 8pm to 6am from Monday to Thursday. Afterward, due to necessitation, she began to work on Friday nights, also. Even though her work hours began at eight o'clock, most nights, she would voluntarily come to our house between 7pm-7:15pm. Unlike the daytime worker, Ms. Night gave my parents medicine, and she also did their laundry. As I recall, Ms. Day said that she did not want to give my parents any medication because she was not licensed for this, and she did not want to violate any public or private laws. Intriguingly, even though Ms. Night did not have any health credentials either, she still gave my mother and father their prescribed drugs.

Although I was unable to find caretakers for my parents twenty-four hours a day and for seven days a week, I came very close to attaining that goal. Additionally, despite the many challenges that we still confronted, to be sure, the status quo had changed radically, all for the better. Meanwhile, my father's weight continued to drop unwaveringly. While my father did not have a large physique, he was not a skinny man either. Rather, I would describe him as someone who was in the middle of both extremes, leaning towards the latter. Thus, with the detection of his cancerous tumors and the ensuing medical treatment for them, once he began losing weight, it was clearly noticeable. One of the chemotherapy's side effects was the lost of taste. Accordingly, he often refused to eat because, in his opinion, most of the food no longer had any flavor. In addition to a significant reduction of his food intake, my father did not consume an adequate amount of water. Even before my mother became confined to a bed, it was common for the both of us to plead with him to drink more water. Although he would get upset with us, because of our recommendations, we never relented. Undoubtedly, his psyche took another blow when my mother was brought home and laid motionless on the bed all day and night. As one can imagine, it must have been mental torture for him to see and to verbally reach out to my prostrate mother, on a daily basis, and there would be no response from her. Instead, he had to regularly watch her in the bed, lying silent and powerless.

Consequently, my father's mind began to deteriorate, similar to the quality of his physical attributes. For instance, prior to his ailment, every evening, just before he went to bed, he made certain to close all the windows in the dining room and in the living room. As long as I can remember, my father did this every day, whether or not the house was hot, cold, lukewarm, chilly, or humid, because he did not want the house's interior to be damaged by falling rain. In the event that one or more persons was occupying both or either of those rooms and/or even if rain was not in the weather forecast, my father religiously screwed down all of the windows. Moreover, before he became ill, he made sure to lock the dining room's two doors. However, due to his declining intellectual and physical strength, when evening time came, and he was about to go to bed, no longer would he perform those two abovementioned chores. On the weekends, Ms. Night was not on duty, and I frequently worried about the security of my parents. Fortunately, on those nights, usually, my brother's son would sleep upstairs with his grandparents. Although he was not a teenager, as yet, his mere presence in the house gave me a sense of relaxation and comfort. Another example of my father's obvious weakening took place during a visit by one of my aunts who lived in St. Thomas. Whilst, my mother's sister, her friend, my father, and I were in the living room talking about various topics, after a while, I noticed that he became silent. Moreover, he seemed to be in a daze and a state of sheer confusion. Our two visitors did not say anything about the drastic change in my father's demeanor. Likewise, I did not comment on it either. However, I am confident that they also became aware of the atmosphere's change. Furthermore, that same night or soon afterwards, I witnessed something that shook me to the core. Usually, after my father went to sleep, I would remain in the living room for a while to watch tv, and I would repeatedly check on my mother to see if she needed anything. In this particular incident, when I went into the bedroom with my father, I asked him if he was okay and whether or not he needed anything before I fell asleep. As was common with him, he said that he was fine. Then, he asked me, "Has your father come home yet?" Stunned, I paused for a few seconds and tried to collect my wits. Then, I said, "My father? Daddy, are you okay? You're my father, remember?" Immediately, he started to laugh and said, "Oh yeah! That's right." Wow. I was totally traumatized, disturbed, and in shock by my father's question. That night, it took me an extra longer period of time to fall asleep, as I frantically made efforts to understand what was going on in the mind of my father.

Around this time, I also noticed that my father began to skip his daily showers. He would say, "Derick, I am not going to bathe today" or "Derick, not today, I don't think I will bathe today." Of course, I never asked him why he chose not to shower. Instead,

I would just let him know that it was okay and ask if he needed me to do anything for him. One time, while I was in the living room and Ms. Day was in the bedroom giving my father his breakfast, she shouted for me to come. When I went to them, she told me that he told her to call me. He was sitting up in the bed and said, "Vomit. Vomit. Derick, I feel like I want to vomit. Go for the bucket. Bring the bucket!" Without missing a beat, I went for a small basin and put it between his legs. Thereafter, I proceeded to rub his back and told him that he is going to be okay. I also informed him that he can always tell Ms. Day to do something for him. I let him know that he did not have to call me to do something for him. Instead, I made sure he understood that Ms. Day was also there to help him. He did not bring up his breakfast that morning thank God. However, when I rubbed his back, it felt as if I was passing my palm across pure bones. This feeling totally dismissed any good emotions that I had, after we all realized that he was not going to vomit. Likewise, one day, my father asked me to help him to go to the bathroom. Unbelievably, each time he attempted to put his foot flat on the floor and begin to walk, the foot trembled, when it got close to the floor, and he could not stand! When he realized what was happening, he began to laugh a little and sat back down on the bed. After a short while, he tried again, I was able to get him to stand on his two feet, and we proceeded to the bathroom. I kept wondering why he was laughing in such a grave situation. Then, I concluded that he had to smile and chuckle because the entire episode with his foot was literally incredible! Imagine, he had reached a stage where he could not stand and balance himself with his own power. At this moment in time, my father would spend fewer and fewer hours in the living room with other family and friends. Once upon a time, he would be there with us for most of the daytime.

Periodically, he would tell us that he was "going in the bedroom to take five" (minutes of sleep). Whereas these breaks were well spaced out initially, eventually, he began to take them more frequently. Additionally, the five minute naps (which were actually a little more than the announced time) later turned out to be much longer.

Long before my father's cancer diagnosis and treatment, he was a person who never showed any indications that he was feeling pain. This habit continued after he became a cancer patient. For example, sometimes, my father would be in the living room, lying on the couch and participating in discussions with relatives and friends. Given that he was no longer taking chemo, it was no secret that he would be having increased pain. At these times, there was no question whether or not he was suffering. We knew this because he would become quiet and turn his face towards the wall. Hence, his back would be exposed to everyone. I noticed that he would also engage in this behavior in the bedroom, after he announced that he was "going to take five." Further, the day that my father's oncologist informed us that he was stopping his chemotherapy, he gave my father a bottle of pills and stated that it was supposed to be used for the pain, which he the doctor emphasized that my father would begin to experience with more frequency and force. Unsurprisingly, my father did not want to take the tablets. Even after it was obvious that he was in pain, and my godmother and/or I asked him if he wanted to take the medication, he would often refuse. However, on one occasion, the pain had to have been so intolerable because, after I had offered it to him, and he rejected it, out of the blue, he said, "Derick, where is the medicine? Where are the pills? Are you going to bring it? Bring it! Bring it!" I swiftly got the drugs, gave them to him, and the pain subsided. Clearly, these were all signs that my father was waning and very, very fast.

Although my father's muscles and awareness were withering away, he was astute enough, one day, to call me and Cletis into the bedroom to talk. He grasped a small blue hand bag and said that it contained our parents' passports, bank passbooks, cash, and other important documents. After emphasizing where he kept the container, he further instructed us to make sure that we used the money to pay the caretakers and to pay other necessary bills. He also reminded us to keep up with payments of the property tax. In a fading voice, he said, "Make sure you all keep up with the land tax, eh. Pay the bills when they come in. Don't let them take your mother's land." For me, this was a very moving, yet enlightening, conversation that my father had with me and Cletis. I sincerely felt this way because, although my father understood that his health was better than my mother's, he was cognizant of the reality that his life was also ending. Thus, before he became incapacitated, like his wife, my father made a conscious decision to try to put the family affairs in order. Around this time, I asked him if I should start to fill out the funeral home forms intended for my mother, which the hospice care physician and director had given me on the day that I enrolled my parents in the program, and he said that I should not. Even though my father, like everyone else, knew my mother was in terrible condition, and that she was presumably dying, he told me to "hold off" on completing the application. Perhaps, he was not ready yet to give up on her and still had a glimmer of hope that she would recover.

These were definitely horrific and dreadful days for me. On the weekends, when the caretakers were off and during the week, when I was the only person at home with my parents, I was split between assisting my mother and nurturing my father. Additionally, because of the tremendous pressure on me, I frequently yearned to return to the states, so that I could get some rest and relaxation. On the other hand, I knew it was important for me to stay in St. Thomas and fill a void as one of my parents' custodians. This feeling of ambivalence haunted me for the rest of August 2011, while I was with my parents, until the moment that I boarded an airplane and headed back to Baltimore. The morning that I left St. Thomas, I could not control my emotions and broke down in the bathroom, crying. This was the second time that I remember reaching such a low state during the phase when both of my parents battled cancer. The first time took place, following a visit to the Schneider hospital to see my mother. On that day, one of her childhood friends went to the medical facility to check on her. Well, later that day, when I was home with my father, I took a rest on a bed just for a short time. As I lied there, my mind drifted to a decades old photograph of my mother and her childhood friend, which I had seen numerous times. Next, the image of my mother in the hospital flashed through my mind. When I thought of the stark difference between how my mother looked in the picture and how she appeared in the hospital, I began to weep uncontrollably. Despite my bawling, I made sure that my father, who was in the living room at the time, did not hear me because I did not want to upset him anymore than he already was. On the second occasion, when I sobbed in the bathroom, shortly before I left the house and headed for the airport, I went to my mother, caressed her body, and spoke to her. She did not respond: physically nor verbally. As in the past, one of the thoughts that swam through my mind was whether or not this would be the last time that I would see her and/or my father alive. Although I regularly pondered this question, on this day, I fled to the bathroom and shed many tears because of my parents' current state. Then, I passed by my father who was lying on his back on a bed in another room. What wounded me the most, at this moment in time, was that, when I waved to my father and told him that I would see him later, he did not look at me. Neither did he reply verbally. My father did not even raise his hand and acknowledge me. Instead, like the day when he was in the living room and had a fundamental change in his behavior, my father just stared into space. He just looked up with a facial expression as if he was in a state of bewilderment and complete disorientation. To be sure, this image of my father was one of several that were seared into my mind, body, and soul.

Once I returned to Baltimore, I did my best to get back into the normal routine of teaching at Morgan State University and being counseled by my psychologist coworker. To be sure, this advisor helped me a great extent during my family crises. Even so, I was still troubled having to give so many identical updates to my stateside associates who were concerned about my parents' welfare. At the same time, I continued to get depressing information about my mother and father, especially the latter. For example, my godmother alerted me that my father was shutting down. She said that it became a regular struggle for her and/or Ms. Day to have my father consume water, apple sauce, pudding, and other foodstuff. On one occasion, Butch called me and said that he had called the house to speak to our father. He said that our father was fighting just to talk. When he had asked him what he ate for lunch, Butch said that our father whispered,

"Souuuuup. Souuuup." The way that my brother had told me over the phone was devastating for me to hear. I knew it had to have been much worse for him because he heard it directly. In addition, originally, my father was very reluctant to get a hospital bed for himself because he felt that he was still well enough to use the normal one. One of the reasons why this first became an issue was because Ms. Day stressed that, with the regular bed, it was hard for her to keep bending over and, then, standing upright, when she was feeding my father. Eventually, he acquiesced, and someone from the hospice came and mounted the hospital bed. Similarly, it was a battle to get my father to start using pampers and to allow Ms. Day to bathe him. Thus, it wasn't until after some coaxing by my godmother and Ms. Day that he began to comply. In my opinion, I think he was embarrassed and humiliated for the following three reasons: he did not want his caretakers see his naked body; he felt powerless, having to use the diapers; and he felt emasculated, having to be restricted to a bed. Definitely, these new measures had to have broken him down psychologically.

After my parents returned to St. Thomas from Puerto Rico, they would be visited periodically by family and friends. Whenever I called home, it was a joy for me to hear the voices of individuals who I had not spoken to in a very long time. In a few instances, I talked to some persons for the very first time. However, I was once told that particular individuals had come to see my father. When I heard the identities of these certain visitors, I knew that the end of my father was not too far away. I was confident that this was the case because, when certain family members were near death, my parents would visit them for the first time. This was the case with my father. Although he had been fighting cancer for the previous six years and would be called on by numerous people throughout that period, when these particular persons came to see him for the first time, because it followed the same modus operandi as my parents, I knew it could only mean what I feared. Shortly thereafter, one night, Cletis called me on the telephone. A few seconds after I picked up the phone, he said, "Daddy gone! Daddy gone!" He did not caution me in advance of the awful news that he was about to give me. Instead, he just blurted out the information. The way that he gave me the message was not a surprise because I knew my brother was not a longwinded person. Additionally, I knew that my father was nearing the end, so I was not in a state of shock, after speaking to my brother. Nevertheless, I was scared and felt helpless. One of the main reasons why I felt this way was because I had never planned a funeral before. I knew that I would get help from family and friends, while I was making funeral arraignments, but I still felt feeble, at the time. Be that as it may, I knew that I would have to be the person who would spearhead the preparations.

My father died on November 19, 2011: my mother's 71st birthday. How ironic is that? Earlier that month, my wife had traveled to St. Croix, U.S. Virgin Islands to be with her mother, who was ailing at the time. While my wife was away, she bought a plane ticket for me to travel to St. Thomas. Prior to my trip, my godmother had given me steps that I would need to follow while making the funeral arrangements. She explained that, first, I would have to speak with the pastor of the Moravian church and find out what day and time she would be available to preside over the day of the funeral service. Then, I would have to go to the Virgin Islands Department of Public Works to inform the government agency of where my father would be buried and to pay for his interment. Next, I would have to visit the funeral home, submit death announcement information for the local media, select a casket, and get other relevant data from the funeral home. Later, I would have to meet with the Moravian church pastor to discuss the funeral booklet and plan the going away observance. Accordingly, a couple days before I left for St. Thomas, I made plans to have someone proctor my classes, and I told my associates about the passing of my father. Once I had made certain that everything was in place in the states, I made the somber journey home. It is one that I was terrified about, but I knew I would have to make eventually.

Once I arrived in St. Thomas, I went straight to my parents' house, as usual, and I went to my mother. She was still not talking to anyone, and she was asleep. As I expected, I suffered an emotional blow when I passed by the room where my father slept. Seeing his clothes and the empty space was tough, so I quickly continued onto the room where my mother was staying. By this time, one of the doctors had placed a catheter inside of her, as they did my father. Because of how quickly my father passed away, once he too became bedridden, he did not have the catheter for a long period of time. Next, my godmother and I reviewed our plans again on how I would arrange the funeral service. Many times in her life, she had to organize funeral arrangements for her family members, so she was very familiar with the procedure and, thus, she was very beneficial to me. My godmother reminded me to speak to the pastor about her availability to officiate the ceremony. After I did this, Cletis, my godmother, and I met with the pastor at the church office, and we planned the funeral. While this meeting was a sad one, there were moments when the three of us were able to laugh, reminiscence, and learn from each other. Then, my godmother and I went to the Public Works Department, and I completed the relevant paper work for my father's burial. Like the conference that we had with the pastor, the time that I spent in the government agency office was marked by humor, learning, and recollection, even though it was a solemn occasion. Additionally, in both instances, the process ran smoothly.

The next step was for my godmother and me to pay a visit to the funeral home. Before we went there, I met with some of my father's relatives in my parents' house, and they provided the names of certain family members who I had to include in the booklet. Once again, this meeting with my family, and the gathering with the funeral director were informative, and they were not as bad as I thought they would have been. The saddest part of being at the establishment was when I had to choose the coffin for my father. On the one hand, I did not want to purchase one that was too cheap. On the other hand, I knew that I had to be sensible because I was working with a limited budget. Before we left the business, the director informed me that I would have to return to the funeral home with my father's burial clothes, the cash to cover the expenses of the funeral, and I would have to proof read the memorial service booklet. My sister in law, Celtis' wife, created the pin on and the other paraphernalia for the death ritual. Thank God it seemed as if everything was falling into place. However, there was one area that still really bothered me. The nagging issue was how I was going to pay for the funeral. Well, over the years, my father and mother had put aside money for days such as these.

It is from these savings that I paid for the memorial service. In addition, because my father was a veteran of the U.S. Army, I knew that he was entitled to some type of military benefits. Hence, while I was still in Baltimore, I began doing research on how I could access and utilize them. Even though I vigorously looked into the matter by speaking to people over the telephone, talking to individuals in person, checking online, and engaging in other activities, I was still getting nowhere. At times, it seemed as if I was spinning in circles, and I was. Then, when I came to St. Thomas, my godmother and I dropped into the Veterans Administration (VA) office on the island. Bingo. Everything that I was looking for and the answers that I pursued were located in the local agency. In addition to giving me a substantial amount of money to pay for the funeral, the military also gave me an American flag and a headstone to install on my father's tomb. After visiting the VA, I could finally breathe a sigh of relief because the cost of my father's funeral was paid in full. Whew!

Butch came to St. Thomas on the day of the viewing of my father at the funeral home. My wife left St. Croix and traveled to St. Thomas one day before the viewing. A day or two before the actual presentation, the funeral director instructed us to return to the establishment, so that we could proof read the funeral booklet. We were also given an opportunity to scrutinize my father, on the day of the display, a few hours earlier than when program was scheduled to begin. After checking the pamphlet for spelling, grammar, and informational mistakes, we uncovered maybe one or two faults. Whatever the amount of errors that was in the brochure, it was not too many. A couple of us also took advantage of the chance to inspect my father before the commencement of the public viewing. Then, the hour for the viewing of my father had arrived. The sacrament was not as bad as I thought it would be. I think that because I examined him in the coffin, before the general public had an opportunity to do so, the sadness of the occasion was lightened. A second reason, why I think the grief of the event was lessened, was because the mood inside the show room reminded me of a family reunion. Thus, the area was filled with much chatter and talk by my father's family and friends. As in the case of the many persons, who visited him when he was confined to the bed at home, at the viewing, I met individuals who I had not seen in several years, and there were persons at the program who I had never met before. A third reason, why the unhappiness of the open casket exhibit was diminished, was because of the orderliness and cheerfulness of the formal program. Led by one of my aunts, the agenda was filled with songs and testimonies that kept numerous of the participants engaged in a positive way. Although the observance for my father was a distressing time, to be sure, it was not as gloomy as I imagined it would have been, primarily, for the three reasons that I listed previously.

Following the formal procedure, those viewers, who had remained until the end of the program, wished me condolences and departed. Some intended to attend the funeral service and burial the next day. However, there were others who did not plan to come to the subsequent day's mass. Either way, I was happy that they were at the viewing, and I appreciated it very much. Once I reached home, as was usually the case, I went straight to my mother and checked on her well-being. That day, Ms. Night volunteered to come to the house extra early and stay with my mother, while I went to the viewing. This was very thoughtful and nice of her. After I had dropped in on my mother, Carol-Ann and I went to my grandmother's house, which was just a few feet away from my parents' own, and we spent the night there with her. Meanwhile, Butch slept in the house with my mother and the caretaker. Similar to the night before my father's viewing, I had an uneasy rest. This was expected because, as one can imagine, I was overwhelmed with a plethora of emotions, such as anxiety, fear, sadness, and panic. One of the thoughts that ran through my mind was whether or not everything would go as planned during memorial service. Although I had secured the necessary pall bearers for the service, and they had all given me their word that they could be relied upon, I still could not help worrying if some participants would be absent and/or if any of them would be tardy.

Finally, morning came, and everyone got dressed to go to the church. Like the day prior, it was difficult for me to leave my mother. Every time that I had to part ways with her was a terrible sensation. However, the day of my father's funeral had to have been one of the worst instances. Hence, just the notion of going to my father's funeral, while my mother remained prostrate in bed-out of sight and out of mind-was soul crushing for me. Of course, she could not ask me where I was going in my suit and tie outfit, and I did not tell her. Nevertheless, once we arrived at the house of worship, my nervousness began to subside. This was the case partly because some of the pall bearers, ushers, and other relevant persons were already in place. In addition, I was greeted by the smiles of parishioners, and this uplifted my spirits greatly.

As a side note, in the fall of 1992, I attended the funeral of one of my dearest cousins. To my surprise, I was an emotional wreck at her memorial service. Ever since the verbal and physical spectacle that I demonstrated that day, I do not hold up well at funerals. Clearly, I do not holler and scream at every one, but, for the most part, I shed an abundance of tears at the somber functions. Well, I surely did the same for my father's funeral. While I knew that the function would be marked by me weeping and sniveling, I did not expect it to occur so fast. Accordingly, once I had gone up to the casket and looked at my father, during the final viewing period, as I returned to my seat, I came apart. Bam! Just like that. Thank God my wife and other relatives and friends were there to console me. One good part about my wailing and sobbing was that it did not last too long. Unlike for my cousin's 1992 funeral, where I was screaming louder than anyone else in the church, the duration for my crying at my father's home going was a relatively short one. One of the reasons why I was so distraught at my father's funeral was because I kept thinking about my mother at home. The image of her in the bed and not in the church is what set off my emotions that fateful day. Moreover, I was never certain whether or not my mother knew that my father had died. This unanswered question most definitely added to my somber mood.

Without a doubt, I was not the only person who was openly crying that day. For example, one of my father's cousins, who visited him regularly, including before he became bedridden, on at least one occasion, left the sanctuary because he was overtaken by mournful emotions. Similarly, other than when Butch-who was one of the pall bearers along with me and Cletis-helped carry the casket in and out of the church, I do not think he was inside the building. Rather, I remember seeing him in the court yard. Most likely, he remained outside because he could not stand to be in the church where our father was laid out in the front with an American flag covering the coffin. When I noticed Cletis, who was sitting in the back row with his wife and daughter, he had his head down. This may have been a sign that he too was distraught. Meanwhile, if there was anyone, who loudly lamented more than me, it was my nephew-Cletis' son. From the time that he was a baby, my nephew spent most of his time with my parents.

They practically loved and nurtured him more than anyone else. Additionally, once my parents were diagnosed with cancer, he instantly became one of their caregivers, and he assisted my father until the end. As a result, on the day of the funeral, my nephew had to be comforted for the entire duration of the service.

The Moravian church's burial ground is located on a hill that is right next to the sanctuary. Consequently, following a well organized and inspirational home going program, the pall bearers and the hearse transported my father down to his final resting spot. Once we reached the bottom of the hill, a few members of the Virgin Islands National Guard (VING) executed a very short ceremony and, then, they gave me the American flag. From the time that I was a youngster, I learned that my father was once a soldier in the U.S. Army, and I admired this wholeheartedly. As a matter of fact, as a small boy, I would wear his dog tags around my neck with great pride and honor. However, I did not know the richness of his military service. While I was knowledgeable of his years of duty and where he was stationed, I was completely unaware that he had surpassed the rank of private (he was discharged as a sergeant) and was a sharp shooter. It is while I was doing research to get information for the funeral booklet that I learned of these two things and other valuable data on his military career. This small part of the memorial service-the segment involving the VING-was moving, yet appreciative, for me. My mood of ambivalence was amplified when the pall bearers carried my father up the small incline and began to place him in the vault. While he was being positioned inside the crypt, and the tomb maker was sealing it, the pastor conducted a short service. Each time I began to feel a little better, my disposition would take a down turn because I would observe the empty tomb, which was adjacent to the one that now held my father. I would become sad because I knew that this adjacent

empty tomb was reserved for my mother. Accordingly, my sentiments were on a roller

coaster, moving back and forth and fluctuating repeatedly on that day, just as they did

on many other previous occasions. As I tried to avoid the thought of my paralyzed and

speechless mother, at home restricted to the bed, I dedicated myself to work even more

towards her recovery and well-being.

Chapter 4

My Mother's Death and Burial

Shortly after my father passed away, a few individuals asked me if I planned to have a repast on the day of the interment. My response in each case was "no." Because I was mostly focusing on the funeral arrangements and my mother's health status, I did not want to take on another project, even in a minor role. Without question, I was already overwhelmed physically and mentally. Nevertheless, some of my relatives did have a small dining out reception among themselves. Meanwhile, one of my father's cousins surprised me and my brothers when he brought a few pans of food to the house. This relative is the same person who consistently visited my father in Puerto Rico, while he was recuperating in and out of the hospital, and when he was on the road to recovery at home in St. Thomas. Prepared by one of the sisters of this particular cousin, the cuisine included fried fish, Johnny cakes, and seasoned rice. This meal was a blessing; it was so delicious and fulfilling; and my brothers and I truly appreciated the gesture. As a matter of fact, there was such a large amount of chow that we had enough to share with others. Unfortunately for my wife, she did not partake in any of the victuals because she had already returned to St. Croix to be with her mother and other family members. After Butch and I separately told our mother good bye, we returned to the U.S. mainland.

When I returned to Baltimore, I was in a bad state, yet I looked forward to returning to St. Thomas, so that I could help out there and be by my mother's bed side. First, however, I had to complete the remaining two and a half weeks of the fall 2011 semester. In the meantime, my emotional state received a boost when, one day, I received a basket of candies and a sympathy card from the students of one of my classes. Several other students and my co-workers also gave me sympathy cards and expressed their condolences to me and my family. These acts were very uplifting for me, and they re-energized my state of mind. Thankfully, the remaining days of the academic term went by quickly and, after I had administered the final exams and submitted the grades, I began making plans to travel again. Accordingly, I flew to St. Thomas in the middle of December, and I stayed there for little more than a month. So here I was again, making an emotional trip to assist in the process of taking care of my mother. As I made the journey, I could not help but think that this would be the first time I would be going to my pace of birth, and I would not see my father. By this time, I had already become accustomed to Cletis picking me up from the airport, as opposed to my father and/or mother, but this time, my stay on the island would be radically different. On this trip, my father would not be alive. On my departure date from Baltimore, as in the past, only two things were favorable: 1. I would see a movie on the air plane and 2. I would have a book to read during the voyage.

Once I had made it to the house, I immediately picked up where I had left off, regarding being a custodian. In addition to the duties, which I performed when I was by myself, now, with the addition of Ms. Day and Ms. Night, I altered my work schedule to some extent. One of the drawbacks of these days was that they were characterized by much tediousness and lethargy. Accordingly, six days a week (Monday through Friday and Sunday), I stirred out of bed around 6:30am and prepared for the arrival of Ms. Day. Once in the house, she would prepare my mother's breakfast, bathe and dress her, and then proceed to feed her. In the beginning, she verbally showed her displeasure whenever Ms. Day was grooming her. On these occasions, my mother would yell, scream, cry, and wail. I believe that because she was paralyzed, her muscles and body were sore. Consequently, every time the care taker lifted her arms, moved her legs, and turned her body, my mother shouted in pain and agony. In many instances, Ms. Day would close the bedroom door, in order to diminish, as much as possible, all the noise that my mother would be making. Every now and then, the care taker would call me and ask me to assist her with making up the bed, holding my mother, or some other thing. In addition to be a care taker, Ms. Day was also a home maker. Thus, she would tidy up the house to some extent. After she had finished tending to my mother and mopping the floor, Ms. Day would listen to the radio and watch television with my mother. Usually, they would both look at soap operas and "The Price Is Right." During these monotonous days, there were two things that I looked forward to. They were the following: 1. I would have enlightening discussions with Ms. Day about local, national, and international news/gossip and 2. Ms. Day, sometimes, would bring treats for me, such as mangoes, kenneps, and other delicacies. Next, shortly before it was time for her to leave, Ms. Day would check on my mother, tell her good bye, and then leave promptly at 2pm.

From time to time, when my godmother came to the house to help take care of my mother, Ms. Day would just be gathering her personal belongings to leave. Once she left, my godmother and I would start our session of taking care of my mother. This phase would be marked by the both of us feeding my mother, singing to her, saying prayers, and doing our best to keep her comfortable. Like Ms. Day, it was very common for my godmother to lavish me with food, and the both of us, most definitely, had our times sharing news/gossip. In some instances, my mother was able to contribute to our discussions and reminisce by saying one or two words. Once my godmother left around 5:30pm, I would keep my mother company, until Ms. Night arrived between 7:00pm and 7:15pm.

Every time that Ms. Night was on duty, I assisted her with the changing of my mother's clothes, the bed sheets, and other things that she asked me to do. Like Ms. Day and my godmother, I also had conversations with the night worker about news/gossip. On a few occasions, she would also bring me some type of food. Without a doubt, the best part of Ms. Night's company was when we would watch movies together. Accordingly, after we had finished tending to my mother, the both of us would go outside and watch movies on television, or mostly, DVDs of African movies that the night worker would bring to the house. Sometimes, if I didn't complete the movies by Friday, she would allow me to keep the DVDs, so that I could watch them in their entirety over the weekend. To be sure, the most depressing part of these dull days was when I would assist Ms. Night with the cleaning, moving, etc. of my mother. To see the looks of pain, anguish, and shallowness on my mother's face either brought tears to my eyes or almost did. By the time I would go to sleep, I would be extremely tired. After sleeping for just a couple hours, I would wake up again and do the exact same things the following day.

Initially, my mother would just lie silently and motionless in the bed for 24 hours a day, 7 days a week. She could do nothing for herself. Periodically, one of her legs would swell to a huge size. Moreover, due to the stroke, all of her fingers were kept bent, and one of her forearms was positioned at a 90 degree angle. Not being able to move herself, she rested on her back constantly, unless Cletis alone (sometimes his wife would assist him), or the caretakers moved her to turn her, change her pampers, or for some other reason. As noted earlier, when I was in St. Thomas, I would assist him and the caretakers with this duty. As I traveled to and from St. Thomas, during my breaks from Morgan, I would get the report that my mother was not speaking. However, one day, Cletis told me that, while he was in the kitchen, our mother yelled, "Cletis!" Totally surprised and caught off guard, he said that he rushed into the bed room to be with her. At some point later, she would stop talking again. Then, she would resume speaking. Like the changes in her leg's size, her ability to talk fluctuated.

On a regular basis, my mother was visited by a staff of the hospice: a nurse, a doctor, a social worker, or a pastor. On some occasions, more than one worker would show up to the house on the same day. Usually, however, they did not all visit on the same day and at the same time. Whenever my mother took in sick with a cold or some other illness, during the day time, at night, and/or on the weekends, and the situation was an emergency, a physician would stop by the house to treat her. During these times, Cletis and I remained in touch with each other over the telephone, and he and/or the tending medical practitioner would give me updates on the status of my mother. To be sure, these were definitely worrying times for me because I was not in St. Thomas, and I could only await word from my godmother, Cletis, or someone else about how my mother was faring.

Every time I came to St. Thomas, I would frequently go to the grocery stores and some other business establishment to purchase necessary supplies for my mother. My shopping list was usually the same, and it included the following items: pudding, jello, cranberry juice, Vaseline, toilet paper, hand towels, tooth paste, gloves, detergent, apple sauce, baby food, seasoning, water, cream of wheat, and soup. I also made sure to buy snacks, already prepared food, bread, cheese, and other foodstuff for myself. In the meantime, one of my aunts, who lived in St. Thomas, on a regular basis, would cook food for me. Her meals included chicken, rice, and vegetables. To be sure, the many edible items that she gave me were a tremendous boost to my physical and mental state. Moreover, my parents and my grandmother were enrolled in the Meals on Wheels program, so most of my mother's food came from this meal plan. Sometimes, I ate some of the things that were sent for my mother. Similarly, my grandmother also gave me some of the victuals that were from the Meals on Wheels program. I used the money from my parents' monetary savings to buy supplies for my mother and father. This included when my wife and I would shop in Baltimore for dresses, pampers, bed pads, and other items for my mother. On some occasions, I would use my own money to buy the goods. Furthermore, when I was in St. Thomas, I often used public transportation and walked whenever I needed to get to a destination. Cletis and my godmother were two other ways that I used to get from one location to the next in St. Thomas. On a few occasions, tensions would mount in the house among my parents' custodians usually over some petty misunderstanding related to the consumption of foodstuff that were bought solely for her, how my mother was cared for, and/or whether or not she was receiving adequate supervision. I despised all of these cases, and they made me sick to my stomach! I could not fathom how my father was deceased, and my mother was fighting to stay alive, yet, trivial matters would take precedence over my mother's welfare. At these times, I almost went crazy! Instead of losing it, I tried to remain focused and to continue to do everything possible that would ensure that my mother would survive and be comfortable.

Likewise, a point of unpleasantness would take place, sometimes, when I had to pay Ms. Day and Ms. Night. Hence, Cletis and I utilized a system whereby I would contact my parents' banker via email, instructing her that Cletis would visit the financial institution and make a withdrawal on a particular day. Most times, he had no problem getting the funds. However, there were times when he would go to the bank, and he would be denied the money because the banker was unavailable, she did not receive my note, the bank adopted a new policy, or some other issue had arisen. Sometimes, he would have to leave the bank, go back to work, and, then, return to the bank on another day. To be sure, it was bad enough that my mother was in such a dire state; however, when I got problems withdrawing money to pay the care takers or to pay some type of bill (for example electricity, phone, or VI property tax), it made the crisis much worse.

When both of my parents were restricted to the house and/or bedridden, they would have visitors in common. This included individuals from the Moravian church and the Lutheran church. Representatives from the former would usually look in on my father and on my mother, since both of my parents attended the church. However, the people, who came from the Lutheran church, mostly, were there to see my mother, since she was still a member of that religious institution. In addition to singing, praying, and reading the Bible, the parishioners also provided my parents with Holy Communion. After my father passed away, Cletis told me that the amount of people who came to the house dropped significantly. For the purposes of clarification, it is important to note that he indicated that my mother still had visitors, but the number was much less than when my father was alive. Nonetheless, he would continue to emphasize that my father's cousin, the one who surprised me and my siblings with food on the day that my father was buried, continued to visit my mother faithfully.

As my mother lied on her back in the bed for one year, then for one and a half years, her health improved and then declined cyclically. Eventually, one of her legs began to swell once more and this time, it did not reduce in size. The hospice physician on call explained to me what was happening to my mother medically, and she said that my mother was dying. She said that she would give her about ten more days to live. For certain, I was horrified by the ominous news. However, I did not accept it entirely because, almost two years earlier, my mother's neurologist had told me and Cletis that my mother had a range of two weeks to six months to live. Moreover, I was also concerned with the dwindling amount of money that was left in my parents' savings account. To be sure, it categorically was shrinking, and my mother's social security benefits were barely enough to pay the caretakers, buy food/medical supplies for my mother, and to pay bills. Once again, I was caught in a quagmire. On the one hand, I did not want my mother to die, yet I did not have enough money to keep her alive. What a dilemma! Simultaneously, I was receiving tremendous pressure from various persons to cut back on the hours of my mother's care takers, utilities, and other expenses. It is at this point that I reached out to a social worker in the Virgin Islands Department of Human Services and to other public and private officials, inquiring what steps I could take to keep my head above water and to keep my mother in the land of the living. For the most part, the persons, who I spoke to, were very helpful, and they provided me with some great ideas on how I could achieve my goals. Immediately, I implemented some of their proposals, including getting an additional custodian at no cost.

Around this time, I was stressing so much that I think I lowered my weight to a level that I had not been in decades. As a result, my cholesterol numbers began to decline because of the reduction of my body weight. I remember my cousin, who lived in Virginia, and other people telling me that, while it was admirable for me to take care of my parents with such commitment, I still needed to make sure that I took care of my own health. Due to the grave financial and mental situation that I was in, at the time, their messages went in one ear and out the next. Once, after I had returned to Baltimore on a Saturday night, my physical appearance was frightening, to say the least. While I knew that I had lost some pounds, I did not realize how much I had shed. Accordingly, when my wife picked me up from the airport and had a good look at me, she refused to allow me to accompany her to church the following morning, because she said I had "looked bad bad." From her perspective, she said that I needed to stay out of public view for a while, until I had regained enough weight to look presentable. Around this time, the frequency of reports about my mother's dilapidated fitness began to intensify. Thus, similar to the period when my father was on his last legs, I was notified that my mother was hardly consuming anything that was given to her. Additionally, the bed sores, which now covered some parts of her bum and heels, increased in size, and they were not healing, as in the past. Meanwhile, blisters also developed on my mother's ears.

Then, one morning a little after 4am, about ten days after the hospice physician's ominous prediction to me about my mother, I received a telephone call from Ms. Night. Once I heard her voice, I knew the inevitable had occurred. She simply stated that my mother had passed on. My mother died on October 10, 2013. Shortly after I hung up the phone, the secretary for the hospice called me to give me the same message and to express her condolences. Thus, after almost one year and eleven months, once again, I had to make arrangements to leave Baltimore and to travel to St. Thomas, in order to make the funeral arrangements for one of my parents. This time around, my wife made the trip with me, and we hit the ground running. Since I had newly made funeral preparations, when I did it for my father, this occasion, I was not as apprehensive and panicky as when I did it the first time. Accordingly, the process was very similar, and it seemed like déjà vu. First, I set up a date to meet with the Moravian pastor, so that we could organize the memorial service. After a funeral date was established, I went to the Virgin Islands Department of Public Works and completed the necessary paper work. Then, I went to the funeral home, provided the director with the pertinent information for the death announcement, which would be sent to the local media, and next I selected a casket. Since my wife was me, during this phase of the planning, my godmother was not with me at all times this time. Instead, because of Carol-Ann' presence, my god mother had a chance to take care of her own personal business and get some rest. Nevertheless, she did assist again throughout the organizing for the rite. For example, she accompanied me when I met the pastor to schedule the service, and she provided me with valuable data for the obituary, especially, since she and my mother were friends and co-workers for many years.

The day of my mother's viewing or the day before it, Butch arrived on St. Thomas. While I am sure that my wife and I went to the funeral home to proof read the funeral booklet, I am not 100% certain if Cletis and Butch were also with us at the time. If we found any mistakes, it was a very small amount. As before, the family was given an opportunity to examine my mother, earlier than the public. Once again, this chance was helpful because it lessened the grief that I experienced at the official display. Akin to my father's exhibit, my mother's viewing was like a mini family reunion, whereby, I met numerous family and friends, some who I had seen recently, and others who I had met for the first time. The following day was the funeral ceremony and, although it was a sad affair, resembling that of my father's, my mother's home going service was still a lively one. For sure, seeing my mother, lying in the casket, was very troublesome for me to witness.

However, I was happy that she was no longer being afflicted. Imagine, for a little more than two years, my mother was positioned on her back, not able to help herself, mostly not able to communicate, and endured abundant days of ache, excessive weight loss, and soreness. She did not even have the wherewithal to ask someone to bring her a glass of water or to instruct somebody to scratch her back. Instead, she usually laid there for all those months nodding, smiling, grimacing, and sighing. While there were days, when she laughed quietly, and, and uttered a few words, for the most part, she was silent, repeated words/phrases that were said to her, and counted from one to one hundred continuously. Moreover, there were times when she would ask someone rub her leg, stating that it was hurting her. However, because of her state of mind, no one knew if her leg was really stinging her, or if she was just talking out of her head. As a result, upon observing my mother in the coffin, I could not help but breathe a sigh of relief. This feeling was not one of joy that my mother was dead. Rather, it was an expression of gratitude that, finally, God had chosen to end my mother's pain and suffering. What an impasse!

The church service proceeded, and it was soon time to bury my mother. Unlike the case with my father, I did not cry at the church service. Initially, I thought this was strange that I did not break down in the sanctuary. Later, upon reflection, I think I did not wail and carry on because I had witnessed firsthand the anguish and torment that my mother endured for several months, so, when she died, as noted earlier, I interpreted it as a time to rejoice, not cry, because she would not be tortured anymore. However, my godmother cried a lot during the ritual. This was expected since she and my mother were such close friends. Additionally, I did not see Butch inside the church. Instead, I noticed him outside in the assembly hall and in the church yard. As with my father's situation, Cletis sat in the back with his wife and daughter, while his son, who cried plenty, was seated with other relatives. Following a service marked by inspirational singing and preaching, it was time for the internment of my mother. Again, Cletis and I served as pall bearers for our mother. This time, Butch was not one because he said his leg was bothering him. Slowly, we filed out of the building and down the incline. Then, we trudged up to the double burial chamber. Observing the tomb maker getting ready to seal the crypt with my mother inside of it and hearing the graveside hymns were two of the lowest points, the saddest feelings, the most gut wrenching moments of my life, thus far. After being a warrior side by side with my parents in their battle against cancer for eight years and four months (June 2005-October 2013), the war was finally over. As I walked down the hill and left the church grounds that morning, my strongest consolation came from the fact that I knew my parents' final resting place would be sleeping beside each other forever. It is the way that they both would have wanted it, and it is the way that it was destined to be.

Epilogue

After I received my PhD in History from Morgan State University on May 16, 2009, I said that being a graduate student and working to achieve the degree was the hardest thing that I had ever done in my life. Well, it truly was, until 2011, when my mother was diagnosed with cancer, and my father's battle with the same disease began heading in a downward direction with full speed. Thus, beginning in 2011, I had to ramp up my efforts in addressing the needs of my parents, and this took a heavy physical and mental toll on me. During the early stages of graduate school at Morgan, one of my professors told the students in class that, for the next few years, our dissertation project will become a part of us. He said that we will dream about it nightly, the stress of the work would cause our blood pressure to rise, and we will become inseparable from it. Using himself as an example, he emphasized that, when he was in our position, he had nightmares regularly about this academic work, his blood pressure rose, and the manner in which he spent his life was tremendously influenced by his research and writing. While I initially gave little credence to his words, I subsequently realized that everything that he told us on that day was true. Well, my experience with my parents having cancer was akin to the dissertation. Accordingly, I had nightmares on a regular basis, involving one or both of my parents. Whereas my blood pressure did not rise, I suffered headaches, dizziness, loss of weight, and mental stress.

Moreover, the idea and medical care of my parents' cancer followed me everywhere that I went. They partly determined where, when, and how I would take vacations, how I would treat myself, my outlook on life, and my overall aura.

Undoubtedly, I could not get away from the subject. Even though I would not be in St. Thomas, sometimes, the trauma was just one phone call away. For example, one Sunday morning, while I was leaving a Baltimore church and walking home, I got a telephone call from my father. Immediately, I started to get alarmed and feared the worse because it was very unusual for him to call me. As long as I can remember, my mother always made the calls to me to find out how was the weather, how I was doing, or for some other reason: big or small. Hence, when I recognized my father's voice on the cell phone, saying, "Derick! Derick!" I almost literally passed out. Nevertheless, the reason why he called was to let me know that an ambulance had come for my mother and had taken her to the emergency room because she had suffered a blood clot in her leg. This incident took place prior to her stroke. It happened during the period when she was supposed to be walking often, in order to prevent such coagulation.

Another time when a phone call demonstrated that, even though I was off Island, it was as if I was still in St. Thomas, occurred, one day, when Cletis called me. Again, a call from him was very unusual because I commonly telephoned him and not the other way around. In the majority of instances, whenever he called me, it was to let me know that there was a problem with a bank transaction, or my mother had fallen ill. Consequently, when I picked up on his voice, my heart began to race, and I became terrified. In this instance, the purpose for him calling me was to ask me if I knew where a certain set of keys was located. Whew! While it was a relief that nothing awful had happened to my mother, it was an unnecessary phone call because he could have asked one of the care takers. This was an example of the insignificant matters that could have been avoided. It was bad enough that I got upset over calls based on emergencies still I had to deal with such trivial issues.

Moreover, as one can imagine, since I was the Power of Attorney for my parents, I had to deal with several family matters, whether I was in St. Thomas or in Baltimore. For example, after my father died, I did a lot of research into areas related to my father's life insurance policies and other business affairs. Sometimes, we learned things in this area indirectly. For instance, one day, Cletis told me that, while he was in an establishment doing his own business, a lady told him that he looked just like our father who had recently passed. Thereafter, she told him that we should check into a certain firm because she was sure that my father was a client of the aforesaid company. Well, I made some calls, based on the data that the lady had given Celtis and before you know it, Bingo. She was correct about my father's relationship with the company, and I was able to attain the funds. Next, I divided the currency equally between me and my siblings because, from the time we were children, my mother always instilled in us that everything that belonged to her and my father should be evenly divided among their three sons.

Despite the tragedy of my parents' illness, the entire experience was, nevertheless, an enlightening and learning period for me. For instance, after my father was diagnosed with cancer in 2005, I became more health conscious. Accordingly, within two years, for the very first time, I took the initiative of getting annual check-ups from a primary care physician. This development included undergoing colonoscopies, prostate exams, physical examinations, and checking my cholesterol. In addition, I have done my best to walk 30-40 minutes daily or do some type of physical activity every day. At the time that my father took in sick, he did not show any overt sings of feeling ill. Neither did he complain of feeling sick, not even a cold. Even with the loss of his weight, no one would have ever believed that cancerous tumors were growing inside of his colon at the time. As a matter of fact, one of his surgeons said that this particular organ may have been targeted eight years prior to the revelation! I think the fact that my father was living his life normally and did not realize that he was a very sick person is one of the main reasons why I changed my diet, began to exercise regularly, and set out to get medical tests often. In sum, my father's case plainly and literally scared the bejesus out of me, so I committed myself to having a healthier lifestyle.

As another example, after I realized the important role of notary publics, shortly after August of 2011, I made plans to become one. Running around the Schneider hospital, traveling throughout St. Thomas, and residing in Baltimore, it seemed that almost everywhere I went, I needed to have something notarized. Once I did get my document(s) stamped, I would always breathe a sigh of relief because the load/pressure on my shoulders was not as heavy as they were earlier. Thus, I began to realize that notary publics serve the general populace sincerely, and they make positive contributions to humanity. It is at that point that I, subsequently, visited the appropriate government office in Baltimore and was certified as a Notary Public. Consequently, I have been able to assist others and bring smiles to their faces just as it had been done to me many times before.

Sometimes, I wonder which was worse for my mother from 2011-2013: the mental ordeal that she endured for those two years or the physical torment during the same period. Since there is no measure that I can use to get a decisive answer, I have tried not to dwell on the question too long and too hard. What I do know, however, is that she suffered. She went through so much both psychologically and in the flesh. For example, soon after her cancer diagnosis, I told the dire news to the Schneider hospital's secretary who was stationed at the front of the oncology center. When I informed her that my mother's fight against the disease would be a difficult one because she was aware of the experiences of cancer patients, and I knew that she could not tolerate chemotherapy, the secretary responded that she agreed wholeheartedly with me. She continued that, many times, while my father was getting the drugs, my mother would be in the lobby wailing and bemoaning, saying that she could no longer bear to see my father agonizing the way that he was. In a later conversation, the staff worker told me that my mother had mentioned to her that she believed my father had given her the disease. As hard as it is to believe, my mother had told the secretary, and she was telling other people that cancer was contagious, and she had gotten it, just like how someone would catch the cold. Clearly, in my opinion, this indicated that my mother had undergone some kind of brain trauma.

A few months into the point, when my mother was bed ridden, the Virgin Islands Government began a project to demolish about five public housing buildings in my parents' immediate neighborhood. One of the edifices was a few steps across the street from where my parents resided. Accordingly, for at least eight hours a day, five days a week (sometimes six) construction workers hammered, sawed, drove bulldozers, shouted, and did numerous other activities less than a stone throw away from my mother's bed. As bad as it was for her to be paralyzed and stretched out in the bed for several months, what was even more terrible was that she had to put up with so much clattering, racketing, and blasting. Of course, most times, she could not verbally complain about the deafening sounds. Instead, she just kept still, gritting her teeth and moaning. After seeing how much beatings and anguish my parents went through, it has definitely put things in perspective for me. Thus, whenever I go to the doctor, to lessen my discomfort, I usually think of when my father was getting bad reactions from chemotherapy and the aches and pains that my mother endured.

In 2016, three years after my mother passed away, I am still scarred mentally from the chapter of my parents' lives when they became cancer patients. When I go into the grocery stores, and I see containers of pudding, jello, baby food, and pampers, I consistently get flashbacks of the times when I would purchase these Items for my ailing parents. Likewise, every now and then, I would get mails for my parents from AARP and other senior citizen programs that they were enrolled in. A simple glance at the address would bring back so many hurtful memories for me. Additionally, when I go into medical facilities, when I see/hear anything about the field of cancer, and when I see people, who have been afflicted with the sickness, my mind gets overloaded and, sometimes, I feel like I want to cry. In some instances, I can and will avoid the signs that result in me reminiscing. However, there are times when I am not able to prevent the occurrence. For instance, countless times, I have been listening to the radio, when all of a sudden, a song will begin to play-such as Luther Vandross' tune "If I Could Dance with My Father Again" or Diana Ross and the Supremes' song- "Some Day We'll

Be Together," and a flood of emotions would gush over my body, soul, and mind. This is all a testament to the reality that, like my dissertation work, my parents' cancer and how I dealt with it will forever be a part of me.

While I took a lot of blows and shed an abundance of tears, during this era of trials and tribulation, never did I ever give up on my parents or leave them to the wolves. Even when my mother was on her death bed, and various individuals urged me to tell her it will be okay if she passes on, I will be fine, just let her go, I wholeheartedly refused to comply. Whenever I needed their affection and care, my parents willingly gave it to me. When I suffered a brain aneurysm and endured brain surgery on March 15, 1986 and March 16, 1986, respectively, my mother and father did not abandon me. Instead, they made sacrifices and did all that was essential, in order to ensure my full recovery. It is like when I was making the funeral arrangements for my father. I asked Butch if he would like to be a pall bearer. Immediately, he said, "Derick, listen, daddy has carried me all my life. Now, it is time for me to carry him. Yes, I will be a pall bearer." Well, once I learned of my father's diagnosis of cancer in 2005 and then my mother's own six years later, my reaction was not to leave them by the wayside. On the contrary, my response was to, as in the words of my brother, "Carry them" as they had done to me for all of my life. As a result, I know that I am a stronger person today, a better individual. Yes, my parents' affliction was the nadir of my life. For certain, it is a period when I had hit rock bottom. Nevertheless, upon hearing of their illness, I made a determined decision to care for them, to hold them, and to nurture them, just as they had done to me. When all is said and done, my wish is that I can also extend showers and blessings of affection to others just as my loving mother and father did to me.